Making Age Just a Number

Making Age Just a Number

A 7-step journey to your
most empowered life

LYNDAL LINKIN

For my boys, Luke, Ben and Sam

Disclaimer
The material in this publication is of the nature of general comment only, and does
not represent professional advice. It is not intended to provide specific guidance for
particular circumstances and it should not be relied on as the basis for any decision
to take action or not take action on any matter which it covers. Readers should obtain
professional advice where appropriate, before making any such decision. To the
maximum extent permitted by law, the author and publisher disclaim all responsibility
and liability to any person, arising directly or indirectly from any person taking or not
taking action based on the information in this publication.

Contents

Introduction

It's right there in front of our eyes. Every day, on social media or the TV we see it. We no longer have to age the way our parents and grandparents did. It is a reality – today we can slow the aging process more than we ever could before. Not only can we look better and feel fitter but our zest for life and sense of purpose can bring so much more joy into our lives as we become older and wiser while still retaining our youth. This is literally the 'old head on young shoulders' we always wanted while still retaining our youthful looks.

Along with all the digitally enhanced images we see however, comes the advertising . . . We're living in an era where the quest to stop aging and look perfect is everything and the advice on how to achieve it is everywhere. There's too much choice and conflicting messaging and it leaves us feeling overwhelmed. Never in history have we been more obsessed with how we look. Never in history have we had so much information overload about how to stay looking young and attractive thrown at us.

With the advancements in creams, procedures and surgery and the new findings in diet and exercise, we can now confidently slow the aging process. The information overload is so overwhelming however, we don't know where to start or what to do. What really works?

We are all looking for the fountain of youth in a jar. Should we buy a cream, a serum or a mask? If we walk into a department store, how do we know which one to buy or how much to spend?

Injectables such as botox and fillers are so popular now and still very misunderstood. Should we use them to prevent getting wrinkles or do they fix the ones we already have? Will they improve our looks without making us look fake or overdone?

Advances in technology mean that non-invasive procedures can defer the need for surgery. In the future, they may even be a replacement. What are they, what do they do and how much do they cost?

I absolutely love the show *Botched*. I watched it from beginning to end during Covid. It's fascinating to watch what people will do to themselves. It is these sorts of horror plastic surgery gone wrong stories that stop people from considering surgery due to fear of pain, long recoveries, scars and no longer looking like themselves.

Then there is diet and exercise. If you type the word 'diet' into Google, there are literally millions of results. Seriously, when and why did food become so confusing? We all know we have to exercise, however when we are so time-poor and exhausted from our normal daily lives, what type of exercise should we fit into our hectic schedules to prevent or even reverse the aging process?

So many questions but with far too many answers to comprehend.

Let me help you. I can guide you through this. Let's put the uncertainty away and find some clarity around what you can do. You can achieve and maintain your anti-aging goals with a lot less effort than you think. My advice in this book will cut through all the noise and simplify what you need to know. You can look better and feel fitter and more energised in 10 years' time than you do right now. Right now, I am definitely fitter than I was 20 years ago, I think I look better too and I definitely have far more life experience and confidence.

It may seem like there is far too much to do and it's all just too hard. Knowledge is power so let me give that to you. If you ignore the bombardment of information and concentrate on what you really need to do, you will see that you don't need to be limited or defined by age. Now is the time to tell yourself that this can become a reality for you. I will simplify the information on what to do; you need to decide you are worth it. Small consistent steps in the right direction can change your life. So let's just stop overthinking everything and concentrate on what you need to start doing. Let's decide right now that you are not going to be defined or limited by your age.

I am sure you are thinking that you feel like you are too old, too overweight, too time-poor, too tired or too something else.

I am here to help you and convince you otherwise. You need to put time aside for yourself. It doesn't matter how hectic your life is. That's it, no excuses.

I have been able to carve time out to achieve my goals – it didn't matter what was going on in my life at the time. I am a mother of three boys. I was a single mother for 14 years with my first son, completed my accounting degree, worked for 12 years in accounting and was the Financial Controller of a German manufacturing company. When I had my next two boys, I started my own finance business. In between accounting and finance, I renovated an old building and turned it into a wedding reception centre and restaurant and after that, sold real estate in the suburbs of Melbourne's inner east.

I am not telling you this to tell you what I have achieved but to let you know that you can still look after yourself amid the craziness of life. We need to learn how to stop letting the storms of life overwhelm us. You will surprise yourself, you just need to know what to do and that will make the difference. While I may not know the challenges you face, I hope by sharing my own life experiences and discoveries over the years you will not only be able to maintain how you look and feel but improve this as you get older.

I was born in the Australian outback in the city of Broken Hill. The climate conditions are very harsh in Broken Hill and the appearance of the people who lived there reflected this. I remember sitting at the table in my grandma's kitchen at the age of six and being absolutely fascinated with the deep lines on her face. My grandma had a hard life. I know now that every line on her face had a story but at that age, I was terrified I was going to end up looking like that.

In that moment my fascination with aging was born and I have spent the rest of my life on a mission to make sure that the lines on my grandma's face didn't end up on mine. It wasn't just the lines on her face, though – it was also the stooped way that she walked and the fact that she never smiled. I remember wondering why she had no energy or zest for life and feeling so sad for her that she didn't. I was very scared of her as well – she was always angry and full of resentment and bitterness. I didn't know it at the time but Grandma taught me that you also age on the inside, when you have given up all hope.

So my anti-aging quest began at the ripe old age of six. And then it happened – I found the answer. That same year I was sitting on the floor watching our black and white TV and a commercial came on. I remember it vividly. A woman waited at the train station for her boyfriend to arrive. He arrived, stepped off the train, they ran into each other's arms and he told her how beautiful she was. The caption came up. It was because of Oil of Ulan cream – it would keep you looking young forever. There it was, all my prayers had been answered. Right then and there I decided, at the age of six, I desperately needed some of that cream.

Well, now I am 55 and my lifelong quest to remain young has worked. I feel healthier and fitter and think I look better than I did at 35. I have tried so many creams, procedures, diets – the list is long. Some things have worked, some haven't. I also know that your passion for life will also determine the aging process.

My hope is that as I share my journey, and the results I have found after years of my own research into becoming ageless, you will see that it really is possible to look and feel younger. Even if you do one thing that improves your confidence, that could be the one thing that encourages you to take another step. It may be a change in your mindset or a small change to your appearance that makes you smile when you look in the mirror.

Ageless means to seemingly not get older and to maintain a youthful appearance. It can also mean to be timeless, dateless and enduring. While I don't think we can look 17 when we are 80, being or becoming ageless is something we pursue. In the not-too-distant future, it may become a medical reality that we truly could cure the underlying causes of aging. This book, however, is about living a happier, healthier and longer life with the information, options and science we have available to us today.

Without question, our appearance on the outside drives how we feel about ourselves on the inside. The very way we walk, the way we carry ourselves, how we talk and dress all reflects how we are currently feeling about ourselves. How we feel about ourselves determines our facial expressions, our conversations and who we outwardly become.

So making the smallest change to how we appear and improving our confidence can have life-changing results. It's time to put yourself first; investing in yourself will not only improve your life, but the lives of those around you.

What to expect in this book

This book is all about the importance of self-care. It is not only about maintaining a youthful appearance, it is also just as important, if not more so, to look after yourself on the inside, to maintain joy and purpose. It is about keeping yourself physically, mentally and emotionally well. As important as this is, many of us pay little attention to it as we are so time-poor.

When we are busy and time-poor, often the first thing we neglect is our self-care. The thing is though, that even dedicating a small amount of time to looking after ourselves can make a significant difference in our ability to function well. Making the time to take care of ourselves changes our mood, makes us feel better, decreases stress levels and ultimately makes us more productive.

This is the book I wish I could have written to myself when I was 30 years old. I have been fascinated with the self-help and personal development world and have literally read hundreds of books and travelled to the States to attend conferences. This is a summary of all the books I have read, the courses I have done, the conferences I have been to and the things I have tried and tested that have worked for me.

While any of these chapters could have a complete book written on them, each chapter is written in a way where you can decide if you would like to do some more work in that particular area. You may already be well into your health and beauty journey and only one or two of the chapters may apply. Or you may want to start from the very beginning and apply my framework which follows this introduction. The framework is a step-by-step process covering all aspects of aging well.

I am not a plastic surgeon writing about the intricacies of surgery or a dermatologist or a nutritionist. I am a realist, hoping that I can help you learn to love and believe in yourself a little more and that you will start to practise self-care to become the very best version of yourself, no matter what age you may be.

What I hope for more than anything else as you read this book, is that you make the decision that you are worth it and you start to take action. Even if it is only the smallest of steps. Just start with one thing.

I love this quote . . .

> The only person you are destined to become is the person you decide to be.
> Ralph Waldo Emerson

So, who do you want to be? Do you want to feel youthful, happy and stress-free? Do you want to feel better about yourself both mentally and physically? Do you want to look better than you did 10 years ago? Do you want to feel stronger and healthier?

Let's get started.

If you have read this book and it has helped you, I would love you to share your journey with me. Send an email to hello@lyndallinkin. com.au. You will be surprised by how inspirational your story, and even the smallest of achievements, can be to myself and to others.

If you would like to follow me on social media – @lyndallinkin – I will be posting on the new developments in this ever-changing industry. I would love you to DM me if something has really helped or resonated with you.

HOW TO USE THIS BOOK

The "Making Age Just a Number" Framework

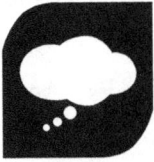

1.
**HONESTY AND GET
YOUR HEAD RIGHT
(SECTION 1)**

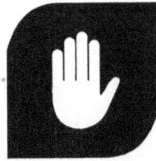

2.
**STOP BEING SLOW, SICK,
STRESSED AND STUPID
(SECTION 1)**

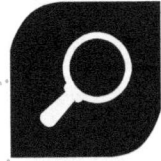

3.
**THE NITTY GRITTY
(SECTION 2)**

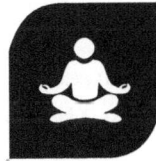

4.
**INSIDE AND OUT
(SECTION 3)**

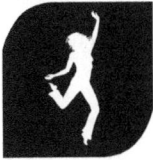

5.
**START MOVING
AND DON'T STOP
(SECTION 4)**

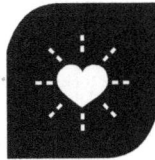

6.
**ME, MYSELF, I – THE FUN STUFF
(SECTION 5)**

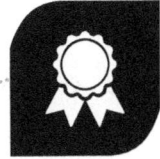

7.
**RECOGNISE YOUR ACHIEVEMENTS
(A SEEMINGLY YOUNGER YOU)**

I am sitting in Byron Bay reading through this manuscript and can see that there is a lot of information here. I have come away to reflect on the book and make sure that I am being truly helpful to my readers. The easiest way to do this is through a framework, or a step-by-step process. I will talk now about the best way to simplify this information and how I have incorporated it into my life.

Use this as a guide to create your long, happy, ageless life. Every human being is on a transformational journey for all of their lives, but how do you want to experience each chapter? Psychologists have long understood that making progress is one of the most important features in an individual's satisfaction and wellbeing, no matter how old you are. Not progressing or getting better is like pain to me, feeling stuck is a horrible feeling.

Step 1 – Honesty and getting your head right

Step 1 is about getting your head into the right space. Don't ever believe that you should have already done or achieved 'something' by now. Should is a terrible word, I always replace it with could. It is perfectly okay to start any journey whenever you want, you don't have to have done it by a certain age. Don't be limited to thinking there is a singular best version of you as there can be many versions of you. This will be different in your lifetime according to your age and experiences. It will change. Your priorities will also change with age and circumstances, and everyone's journey is different.

I always hated the question *'What do you want to be when you grow up?'* Not only did I not know, I felt resentful that I was being made to feel like I should. How do I know? I am not grown up yet.

I hope I never really 'grow up' and lose the curiosity I had as a child. Curiosity drives everything we do – it makes life interesting and fun.

Getting your head right and being honest with yourself is step 1 because your behaviour and actions are directly related to your emotions. What is it you need in your life the most right now? Listen to your gut and deal with one particular thing at a time. Promise yourself to commit to taking the action that is required. I am speaking from experience – if I am not mentally prepared, I will fail, every single time. You need to identify the strong emotional connection to what you are trying to achieve that will keep you on your course.

Step 2 – Stop being slow, sick, stressed and stupid

Start meditating. Give yourself 15 mins every morning before the day starts. This is outlined in Chapter 5. It doesn't have to be hard, it's all about you and finding a state of mind that helps you make the right decisions for yourself moving forward. It can be quite a personal thing when finding the meditation that works for you. Experiment by trying a couple of the guided meditations on YouTube and find one that you are not only comfortable with but that you love.

I love Emily Fletcher. Her meditations are a great place to start. She summarises its benefits by saying that if you don't meditate you will be slower, sicker, stressed and make more stupid decisions. I have found this to be absolutely true and feel noticeably more stressed and unfocused if I don't meditate.

Step 3 – The nitty gritty

Okay, so now you have a strong emotional connection to and know what you want to achieve at this stage in your life and you are highly focused on it because you are meditating every day, you are ready to take action.

The mental resilience you are building will teach you how to be consistent and is something you have to work on every single day. When you become mentally strong enough to be consistent, a great day turns into a great week, a great month, a great year and ultimately a great life. I explain in Chapter 6, it is only consistent, small behaviour changes over long periods of time that will change your world. When you prove to yourself that you can stay the course, something inside of you changes and this is where self-belief and confidence begins.

Step 4 – Inside and out

I think one of the most used cliches of all time is 'you are what you eat'. There is a reason for that – you are, inside and out. Anything you put in your mouth will have an effect on your wellbeing, both mentally and physically. When you are meditating regularly you will start to be more considered about the food you are eating. You will make better, more conscious choices. You will drink more water. You will be more aware of when you are making bad choices and why. You will start to look for the foods that will nourish you.

When you begin to change your relationship with food and see it as a source of nutrition and something to love rather than the enemy, it can be extremely freeing. As you choose beautiful

healthy foods instead of the processed type of food imperson-
ators, these types of choices over time will help your health and
self-confidence skyrocket and increase your longevity.

Step 5 - Start moving and don't stop

You have a definite focus on the right goal and you are feeding your
mind and body with not only the right nutrition but the right information. You are focused. You are starting to feel really good about
life. Next step is to bring it up a level and start feeling awesome.
Exercise is just the bomb, especially resistance training. If you are
a woman my age and you haven't started some sort of resistance
training yet, go immediately and join a gym. Do not pass GO, do
not collect $200 – straight to the gym and start strength training.

Step 6 - Me, myself, I - the fun stuff

When I say 'the fun stuff' I am referring to the things that give
us the instant results, like a great serum, botox, laser treatment
or even plastic surgery. It may be that trip of a lifetime you have
always wanted to take, a change in your career or relationship. The
reason I have made this step number 6 is because, in general we
are more likely to spend money on ourselves or make big changes
in our lives when we start to have a stronger sense of self-worth.
Our self-worth increases and we see ourselves through different
eyes when we keep promises to ourselves and our self-confidence
skyrockets. When you prove to yourself that you can be consistent,
stick to the nitty gritty and take the required actions to achieve
a goal, no matter how small, this will automatically happen.

You have stopped sabotaging yourself and you start to feel like you can do anything. Achievements will make you want to invest in yourself even further.

Step 7 – Recognise your achievements

Taking the time to recognise your successes, no matter how small, helps you to believe that you are worthy of your own approval and creates the positive emotions of self-respect and confidence. It has a cumulative effect, or the 'snowball effect' as discussed in Chapter 6, that contributes to psychological wellbeing, happiness and increased resilience.

If you never acknowledge your accomplishments how do you build confidence, and where do you find the courage to reach for the next important dream or goal? Acknowledging your achievements is a powerful form of self-care that gives you the internal belief you are growing as an individual and that you can do anything you put your mind to – it encourages you to take repeated action, which is everything.

Section 1

Brain health is better than botox

Nourishing and nurturing our minds will absolutely slow down the aging process. This is more important now than ever before because of the amount of information being thrown at us. Our brains are being shaped unwittingly and it is creating enormous challenges to our mental wellbeing.

There are ways, however, that we can take control back of our minds and our emotions, to find happiness and meaning that makes us want to chase that life worth living. Changes in the brain can happen very quickly when you start to move your focus. It is true that if you nourish your mind you can truly change your world, no matter how old you are.

Chapter 1

A sense of wellbeing and happiness

I start with this because we are not going to look good on the outside if we don't feel good on the inside. For many, as we age, life has worn us down. You can see that when you look into someone's eyes and see their soul. Stress, heartbreak, disappointment, resentment, regret and more have taken over, have won.

Some, however, seem so much younger than their age. Their eyes have a glint in them, their walk has a spring in it, they are carefree, loving life and still have a sense of joy and fun. Understanding happiness is probably one of the most important things we can do for longevity. What is the point of looking good and staying young if we are not enjoying our lives? It is very empowering to know that we can work on our happiness.

Happiness has now become a field of scientific research. Happy people are healthier, have a better immune function and have less heart disease. There is also evidence to show that happier people have great mental health and can live up to ten years longer.

A couple of my favourite books on this subject are the Dalai Lama's *The Art of Happiness* and *The Happiness Advantage* by Shawn Achor. They explain that happiness is something that we need to take responsibility for and work on and not something that just happens to us. Learning that we do not have to be victims and can control our responses to what happens to us is life-changing. We can train in happiness the same way we can train in any other skill. You don't need to be lucky or wait for the day when something might happen or fall into place the way you expect it to.

We all have our own ideas about what happiness is. Many see it as a destination. For example, when I achieve a certain outcome, maybe it's money, travel or love, I will be happy. The destination, however, is ever changing. A lot of us tie happiness to our goals – we have the if-then version of happiness. I will only be happy if I get that but when you get to that place you are not satisfied, there is always something else. We get far too caught up in the way we think things should be instead of appreciating what they are and what we already have and have already achieved. The if-then model can therefore be a format to make us unhappy.

We generally regulate our emotions and seek happiness with short-term fixes, such as wine and overeating. Maybe your heart has been broken and you take a bottle of wine over to your girlfriend's house to feel better and then the next morning you feel even worse! You can, however, learn to regulate your emotions without these short-term fixes that over time will be harmful.

In some way, shape or form, our entire life is a quest to be happy. Happiness is not an emotion, it is a state of mind. It is something that can be practised and learned. Joy, fun, excitement, pain, anger and fear are all emotions that come and go. Our state of wellbeing and happiness, however, is what we come back to after the fluctuations in these emotions have gone and it is something that we can work on. We have a certain baseline of happiness and depending on what is going on in our lives, we can go off this set-point as good and bad things will happen to us. Successes may result in a temporary feeling of elation or tragedy may send us into a period of depression but sooner or later our level of happiness falls back to our baseline. So what determines our baseline and how do we raise it to a higher level? The following points will help to raise your natural level of baseline happiness regardless of the highs and lows you are going through. These are long-term strategies rather than the instant gratifications we usually look for.

Do you really care about what that person is doing on Facebook?

That is not an invite to pick up your phone and check your socials, by the way.

Constantly comparing yourself to others can make you feel like a failure no matter how successful you really are. There will always be someone who has more money or material things than you or who seems happier on the outside. Remember, you don't know what is truly going on in people's lives. This is harder than ever to do now in the age of social media where we are bombarded with beautiful happy faces, people with gorgeous bodies, amazing homes and incredible holidays.

Our feeling of contentment is strongly influenced by how we compare ourselves to others. Spend a day away from social media to give yourself a break from these types of comparisons. At the end of the day, check in with how you are feeling. Do you feel better? If so, make it a habit to be aware of when you are comparing yourself to others and if it is making you feel bad about yourself.

> Comparison is the death of joy.
> Mark Twain

What is happening to you right now?

Are you worrying about something that might happen but probably won't? Are you feeling angry about something that happened in the past? Stop. Breathe. I bet right now you are okay – more than okay. This is something, however, that you have to actively be aware of and choose to do.

There is an enormous amount of talk about living in 'the now' across personal development platforms because in this crazy world we really need to take stock, slow down and take back control of the never-ending monkey chatter going on in our brains.

The only way we can experience happiness is to be present. Anger, regret and sadness are all emotions that are a result of something that has happened to us in the past. Panic, worry and lack of control all relate to the future. The only place true happiness and contentment can exist is right now. Philosophers and religions all teach this same theory in many different ways.

We need to learn a calmness of mind and how to simply be right now. This is learnt through the consistent practice of meditation. One of the most significant ways you can raise your baseline of happiness is with meditation. Chapter 5 is dedicated to meditation but it is also important to mention it here. It will help you reduce stress, improve happiness and live longer. It is a proven fact that minutes after meditating we experience calm and contentment.

Practising meditation doesn't mean you have to be all Zen or live an unrealistic existence. It means including it in your life for 15 minutes daily and there are plenty of apps available to help you. It is a non-negotiable practice – you need to do it every day as its benefits compound over time. It will reduce stress and make you a more productive and an all-round better person. It will drastically improve your baseline of happiness if practised consistently.

The Dalai Lama nails it when he says:

As long as there is a lack of the inner discipline that brings calmness of mind, no matter what external facilities or conditions you have, they will never give you the feeling of joy or happiness that you are seeking. On the other hand, if you possess this inner quality, a calmness of mind, a degree of stability within, then even if you lack various external facilities that you would normally consider necessary for happiness, it is still possible to live a happy joyful life.

Just let go

A specialist publication of the *British Medical Journal* showed that people who constantly feel anger are likely to age more quickly. Resentment and anger have long been associated with a whole host of long-term health problems.

The constant flood of stress chemicals and metabolic changes in the body that accompany feelings of anger can lead to high blood pressure, headaches, digestion problems and skin problems such as eczema, asthma, depression, heart disease and can cause heart attacks and strokes.

Releasing resentment and embracing forgiveness is probably one of the most important skills you can learn to achieve happiness. Letting go of resentment is one of the hardest things to do but it is one of the most powerful in setting our hearts free.

There is a famous saying that goes:

Resentment is like taking poison and waiting for the other person to die.
Nelson Mandela

The only person suffering from the negative energy that you are holding on to is you, not the offender. This does not mean that how they treated you was okay, it means that if you can understand this very powerful concept you can release the negative energy from your heart and move on with your life. Hard to do, but an extremely emancipating practice.

And now for something probably even more powerful – self-forgiveness. Recently the University of Hertfordshire in the UK did a study on the things that create happiness and satisfaction for people. The number one predictor of happiness and how satisfied you would be was self-acceptance. So, we need to start learning how to be kind to ourselves. To accept that we will make mistakes and that not one person on this planet is perfect. Do you like yourself? Do you show kindness, consideration and love to yourself? Have you given up all guilt that you may be feeling? Guilt is a good short-term emotion, as when we hurt someone we acknowledge our mistake by feeling guilty. It's a way of demonstrating empathy, regret and understanding. But then you need to forgive yourself and move on from the guilt as residual guilt is extremely self-destructive. Learn from your mistake and move on. This is far easier said than done, but extraordinarily important for your long-term happiness.

Try a little tenderness

Science proves that performing acts of kindness is beneficial for all of the people involved. When you do a good deed or someone does something nice for you, your body releases the feel-good hormones like serotonin and oxytocin. This reduces anxiety, makes you feel calmer and increases happiness, too.

Be generous, volunteer, be kind to strangers and be friendly. Little acts of kindness can make a big difference and really boost your mood. Do you remember when a person showed you kindness when you least expected it? How do you feel now when you think of that person? Heart-warming, isn't it? A smile automatically comes to your face.

I remember when my youngest boy Sam was only four years old and we were staying at the beach for Easter. Of all the things we did with our kids, the Easter egg hunts were one of the things I enjoyed the most. We would hide eggs in so many different shapes and sizes in the front garden and it would take the kids hours to find them all. Then while I kept the kids distracted, my husband Gary would hide the same eggs in the backyard and we would do it all again. So much joy!

One Easter, my parents came down to visit us for lunch. Sam answered the door to them, ran to his bedroom, brought out his biggest egg and gave it to them. This was such a generous and kind thing to do in his four-year-old world. My three boys are all kind, thoughtful and caring. Of all my achievements, this is what I am the most proud of because it has made me feel that somewhere along the way I have done something right. It is my greatest joy and strongest source of happiness.

Now try a little thankfulness

This is another very powerful subject that has become an extremely popular topic and there are very strong reasons why. While you are feeling grateful it is impossible to feel angry, anxious or sad at the same time.

My parents were very strong on gratefulness. The worst thing you could be described as was an 'ungrateful kid'. It is something you are definitely taught and can learn through practice. There is so much truth in it. If two children were to receive the same toy, one threw it on the ground and the other showed extreme gratitude, which one is going to grow into the happier adult?

Happiness is an internal feeling and gratitude plays a large part in this. Gratitude is not only about thinking positively and ignoring the negative aspects of our lives. The best way to practise gratitude is to think about even the smallest things that we are grateful for in our lives first thing when we wake up. A daily gratefulness journal can be very powerful. It changes the perspective in our day. You can notice that there are still simple things to be thankful for even if you are experiencing a very difficult time in your life. It is easy to notice large things like a promotion but what about a pay rise and small things like a warm bed to sleep in. Maybe you like the way your hair looks today. It doesn't matter, it is the daily practice and gradual shift in your perspective over time that makes an enormous difference in your life.

Perfectionism only causes pain

This is something I have always struggled with. It can be debilitating as you never ever feel like you have achieved something.

People with perfectionism hold themselves to impossibly high standards. They think what they do is never good enough. They set ridiculously high goals and when they don't achieve them, they start beating themselves up. Some people mistakenly believe that perfectionism is a healthy motivator, but that's not the case. Perfectionism can make you feel unhappy with your life and interfere with your wellbeing as you do not meet the expectations you set for yourself. Embrace failure because this is how we accelerate learning, stop trying to control a world that you cannot control, stop putting so much pressure on yourself, be aware when you are doing this by looking back at what you have already achieved.

The damaged heart

No one lives without suffering and loss. This does not eliminate the inevitable suffering that comes from loss, but it does reduce it when we understand that we are not alone. We all struggle when dealing with pain in our lives. It might be an agonising experience such as the death of a loved one or the ending of a romantic relationship. Accepting our suffering as a natural fact of human existence and courageously facing it head on is the best way to deal with it. Superficially treating it with alcohol or drugs certainly eases the pain for a while but will not help in the long term.

Try not to judge the experience as good or bad. Trying to make sense of bad things will stop you from returning to a sense of wellbeing. Often there is no explanation why things happen the way they do. In time, once the pain has lifted, you may view the experience as a journey of self-discovery and personal growth. Happiness doesn't mean you ignore pain, it means as you grow and become stronger and better at dealing with pain and uncertainty, your baseline rises.

> Character cannot be developed in ease and quiet.
> Only through experience of trial and suffering can the soul be strengthened, ambition inspired, and success achieved.
> Helen Keller

The yearning for another

There is no avoiding it, our happiness will be strongly determined by the person we choose to spend our life with. While we would like to believe that our happiness can be found solely within us, in the case of a relationship we give up the power of our happiness to someone else. That is scary! It is important to make sure your life partner shares the same values as you while you go through your life journey together because the level of satisfaction in our relationship can increase our life expectancy.

There is an amazing TED talk by Robert Waldinger that has had 38 million views and has been transcribed into 45 different languages. He discusses the longest study ever done into happiness at Harvard over 80 years.

Those who kept warm relationships got to live longer and happier and the loners often died earlier. 'Loneliness kills,' he said. 'It's as powerful as smoking or alcoholism.'

The study showed that the role of genetics and long-lived ancestors proved less important to longevity than the level of satisfaction with relationships in midlife which is now recognised as a good predictor of healthy aging. If your relationship is not working for you, it might be time to have a look at it – it seems your longer life depends on it.

Is there is a particular area in your life that you need to work on to increase your baseline of happiness? Do you need to forgive someone or forgive yourself? Are you constantly comparing yourself to others? Could you be more grateful even for the smallest things? Do you need to embrace imperfection and not be scared of failure? Have you truly faced up to something that has broken your heart? Start taking the smallest of steps every day and then watch how, over time, your baseline of happiness lifts and you start to appreciate and love your life so much more. It will make life worth living for so much longer . . .

Chapter 2

A sense of purpose and meaning

Eighty years ago, a psychologist named Victor Frankl stood up to Sigmund Freud. He said that the primary desire of every person was to experience a deep sense of meaning, and when they couldn't find meaning they numbed themselves with pleasure.

The topic of meaning has also been made extremely popular in the business and personal development world by Simon Sinek. His book *Start with Why* (and TED talk of the same title) is one of the most popular books of all time.

But how does it relate to aging?

A happy life is generally one filled with stability, pleasure, enjoyment and positive emotions. Another component to living a fully rounded life is to live with meaning, purpose and service. Without this, we can give up and feel that there is no point. It is a fact that a lack of purpose predicts an early death. People in their 60s with low purpose in life are twice as likely to die within five years as those with a purpose, with a sense that their life is headed in a particular direction, for a reason. The two most vulnerable times in a person's life are the first 12 months after birth and the year following retirement. In fact, you have probably heard stories about perfectly healthy people who died shortly after they retired from a lifelong career. Some researchers suspect that for these people, the end of their career also signified the end of their purpose in life, which affected their health and wellbeing.

In a study by Dan Buettner on Blue Zones (communities in the world in which people are more likely to live past 100) which identified the factors that most centenarians share, one of them was a strong sense of purpose. In 2014, researchers used data that found 'having a purpose in life appears to widely buffer against mortality risk across the adult years'.

One of the main reasons purpose is important to us is because it has a huge impact on how we view ourselves. Our self-belief and our self-talk are highly influenced by what we feel we bring to the world. Your identity is intrinsically linked with your sense of purpose in life.

Purpose can guide life decisions, influence behaviour, shape goals, offer a sense of direction and create meaning. For some people, purpose is connected to meaningful, satisfying work. For others, their purpose lies in their responsibilities to their family or friends. Others seek meaning through spirituality or religious beliefs.

Purpose, like happiness, is a mindset. It is a choice to live a life that matters. True purpose is about recognising your own gifts and using them to contribute to the world. These gifts could be as large as Elon Musk founding SpaceX or as simple as helping a friend solve a problem. Perhaps it is bringing more joy into the lives of those around you. All are equally valid.

It is important to recognise that your purpose will change over the course of your life. All the decisions I have made and my major purpose in life since I was 20 years old have been to give my boys the best lives and opportunities I possibly could. Now they don't need me as much any more, my focus and purpose can change.

Defining purpose and why we need it in our lives is the easy part. Working out what your purpose is can be the hard part but it is never too late to find a purpose in life. So how do we find our purpose? Your purpose is your passion in life, it is what gives you energy. It is the reason to jump out of bed in the morning. It is the very way we feel alive on the inside.

One of my very favorite authors, Andrew Griffiths, explains it this way in his book *The Me Myth*:

> It's like someone has turned on their button and given them an injection of energy. It is the wonderful side of being human. There is no rhyme or reason to it but everyone has that one special thing that makes them light up like a Christmas tree. When they are in this passionate zone they become a different person. Passion is the fuel of life and the more we have the more we love our lives, no matter what we have to deal with.

Living on purpose feels alive, clear, and authentic. You may also experience 'flow', which is a state of total absorption in which time seems to disappear and you feel content and fulfilled. It is having the courage to live a life true to yourself and not the life that others expect of you.

You can see it when people are living a life true to themselves. I have an Australian Post delivery driver who comes to my house more times than not now that I am a shopping online expert because of Covid. He speeds up my driveway in his van and toots the horn. He jumps out of the van with the biggest smile and starts talking to me in broken English as his main language is Chinese. He usually tells me something and laughs and even though I never understand what he says, I laugh and smile back too. It's fantastic. He then jumps back in his van and says, 'See you tomorrow!' (I understand that much) and waves. He has such great joy for life and it's infectious. He doesn't even know it but he makes me smile on the inside every time I hear him toot the horn and I always wonder how he gets so much enjoyment from a job that I know I would find menial.

So now we know that purpose is fundamental to extending our lives, how do you work out what your one special thing is at this point in your life? If you are not currently passionate about what you are doing it might be time to start thinking about what's next for you or how you can look at including passion in your life and to start living with some purpose and meaning.

Amazon lists over 150,000 books that reference how you can live with purpose. Passion and purpose are in motivational books, TED talks and discussed at length by motivational speakers all over the internet. It can be a little confusing so I will try and simplify it.

There is a TED talk by Richard Leider that is an excellent summary of purpose:

Gifts + Values + Passion = Calling (Purpose)

Purpose is how you relate to others in the world, it is how you share your talents. It is about recognising your own gifts and using them to contribute to the world. The gifts we choose to use will be decided by what we value most in life.

The next part of the equation is where you need to be honest with yourself about what values are the most important to you. You may have many values but you need to prioritise those that have the most meaning to you because ultimately our behaviour is driven by our strongest values. At this point in my life, my most important values are Freedom, Growth, Adventure and Inner Harmony. They are so strong that I am very aware if I am doing something that doesn't meet these values and I adjust my behaviour accordingly. When you are very aware of your inner values it can create discord if something gets in their way. It can also cause conflict with your partner if your values are not in alignment. For example, you may have respect high on your list of values but your partner does not, or your definition of the value may vary.

Sometimes, people talk to me about the fact that their lives haven't turned out the way they thought they would – they don't like their jobs or their partners and everything in their life has flatlined. I smile and ask them, 'Well – who are you at this stage of your life?' They give me a strange look, but after the question has registered and the discussion continues, it is not long before they realise that their lives have totally veered off track from the values that are at the very core of their being. Before they move forward with the next part of their lives, they need to truly assess this.

The final part of the Purpose equation is passion. Passion cannot be found in your head because it lives in your heart. No matter how hard you try, you cannot figure out your passion by thinking about it. You need to take action and feel it on the inside. You need to get out of your head and sometimes your comfort zone and physically do what you have been thinking about and see how it makes you feel. You can't rationalise passion. It's not going to turn up unless you get out there and find it. Or maybe you just need to remember the last time you felt alive on the inside, who you were with and what you were doing.

Be honest about what your gifts are and don't be modest, self-deprecating or put yourself down – we all have gifts. Be honest about what your values are and when you are doing this, make sure you are following your dreams, not the dreams of others. Be aware of or try to remember the last time that you lit up on the inside – sit up and take notice, as this is your true passion. If you haven't found it yet, get out there and try something new and see how it makes you feel.

This is one of my very favourite quotes of all time:

> Our deepest fear is not that we are inadequate. Our deepest fear is that we are powerful beyond measure. It is our light, not our darkness that most frightens us. We ask ourselves, 'Who am I to be brilliant, gorgeous, talented, fabulous?' Actually, who are you not to be?
> Marianne Williamson

When you understand your gifts, your values and your passion, your purpose will start to become clearer. Whatever it is, keep it close to your heart. If you haven't quite worked it out yet, don't worry, open your heart and be open to all the joy and possibilities that living with purpose can bring. Be totally honest with yourself and don't ignore your dreams, whether they be big or small. Get excited about life again and you will feel so much younger.

Chapter 3

A sense of adventure

The next component of living our best and longest lives is to include a wide range of experiences, be they good or bad. It is having the courage to challenge yourself. It is bringing the element of surprise and unknown into our lives through adventure. The experiences could be happy or meaningful or they could be unpleasant but without a wide range of emotions and without any level of uncertainty our lives become boring and monotonous. Some of us are living generally happy and meaningful lives but are bored out of our brains. Does this need for adventure diminish as we age? I hope not – it keeps us feeling alive.

Life is either a daring adventure or it is nothing at all.
Helen Keller

I ran around like a wild thing growing up in Broken Hill. Life was fantastic, you had such a sense of freedom. Such a sense of adventure. There were no locked doors and we had to be outside all the time. As soon as *Sesame Street* finished, we were out the door. None of this inside stuff – it was so liberating. We would ride our bikes everywhere and I would get into trouble with my parents when I pushed the adventure boundaries a little too far. Life was an absolute hoot. Lots of red dirt, our bikes, our friends and our adventures. Every day was a surprise, we didn't know what the day would bring and that is why it was so exciting.

I think this sense of adventure as a child has taught me to take risks as an adult. Be courageous and try new things. And really, what is life without adventure? Do we lose this as we age? When someone has a glint in their eyes and a cheeky smile, they look 10 years younger. They look alive. It is obvious that they are still enjoying life and everything it has to offer.

Risk can be scary, but we're more likely to regret the things we did not take a chance on than things that we did. The major regrets of the elderly are the things they didn't take a risk doing. The adventures they didn't take, not travelling, not taking career chances, not chasing their dreams or the love of their life who got away because they didn't have the courage to express their feelings.

I am going to tell you a story now that I have been asked to recount many times. It is a great example of adventure as I think I went through every single emotion possible in one day.

When my two younger boys, Ben and Sam, were seven and five, my husband Gary and I were discussing where we could go on an overseas holiday that the whole family, adults and kids, would enjoy. After hours of discussion we decided on Hong Kong as a destination rather than a stopover. I am so glad we did as Hong Kong was amazing.

The kids loved it! We went to Disneyland, Ocean Park (which is the best theme park I have ever been to), we sailed on Victoria Harbour, went to Macau, saw the Hong Kong skyline light show every night, went to Victoria Peak and stayed in beautiful accommodation with a rooftop pool overlooking Kowloon Bay. It was brilliant, although I think the kids enjoyed the all-you-can-eat breakfast the most.

Before we went, when Gary told one of his clients where we were going, she almost jumped out of her chair and said that she went there every year and that we MUST visit Shenzhen while we were in Hong Kong to go shopping. Shenzhen is a Communist city where East meets West for the purposes of manufacturing. It grew from a small town of 39,000 in 1980 to a vertical city of 20,000,000 in 2000. It is where all the labels are made, Prada, Chanel, Dior, Gucci and so on. You could buy the real deal for approximately a tenth of the price. For example, a $4000 Prada handbag would cost $400. Okay, so now I was REALLY excited about going to Hong Kong.

About four days into the trip, I couldn't wait any longer, I had to go. But it was proving more difficult than we thought to get to Shenzhen. It required visas and we also didn't think it was a good idea to take the kids. We decided that it was best if Gary stayed at the hotel and I went with a small guided group of about 16 people.

It was an early start the next day. We were leaving at 6am which shows how keen I was as I just do not get up that early on holidays. The books we had read pushed the point to be extremely careful of pickpockets so Gary suggested I wear a zipped waist pack under my clothes. He put in the Visa card for me which works anywhere in China and a small amount of cash.

We met in the foyer and everyone was with their partner or husband except for me. This made me a little nervous, but I just had to keep my eyes on the prize. One lady was from Texas and this was her third trip back. She had a huge list of all the things her friends and family wanted back home.

We had supposedly paid for a first-class train trip but when we got on the train it was the same as being on a Melbourne train in the 1980s. The train was packed, however we were allocated seats. It was going to take approximately 90 mins. It was one of the strangest train trips I have been on. Hong Kong is a vertical city and so is Shenzhen. For the full 90-minute trip, the landscape was wall to wall skyscrapers. I kept waiting for them to stop and for the countryside to start, which didn't happen. Land is certainly precious there – I think we take this for granted in Oz.

Finally, we got there and we had to hand everything over to our guide – phones, passports, everything, and we would not get them back until we left Communist China. Now this made me very nervous and quite afraid. I didn't want to hand over my passport or my ability to communicate. Anyway, on we went, time for the minibus.

Unbeknown to me, the first part of the trip was a guided tour around Shenzhen for a couple of hours. As interesting as this was . . . OMG, could you please just take me to the loot! The guide told us that the Chinese are known for eating anything and everything, and that this was actually true. We then stopped at a local restaurant for lunch, and do you think I was going to eat anything now? Nope, not a chance, didn't eat a thing. One of the meals looked like it was crawling with bugs. On the way back to the bus, I saw a beggar sitting on the ground with half of his body mutilated from burns. The guide explained this happened during a manufacturing accident. It was absolutely horrendous.

Finally, we came to a factory. We got off the bus, they opened a huge steel roller door, we walked in and there it all was. I couldn't believe what I was seeing – handbags, watches, sunglasses, clothes, the real deal – I was in heaven. I spent the next couple of hours blissfully choosing as much as I thought I could possibly get into our suitcases and putting it on to the counter ready to purchase.

Okay, let's pay for this stuff and get out of here, I thought. The sales assistant tallied how much I owed and I reached into my waist wallet for my Visa. I pulled out the card and looked at it in disbelief.

Gary had not packed the Visa . . . he had put in the RACV card which was exactly the same colour.

To this day, I am not exactly sure why he even brought the RACV insurance card to Hong Kong as it was not something we would really need there. I couldn't speak, I was in shock. As the others on the tour realised what had happened, they couldn't believe it either. One of the Texans started laughing out loud, telling me how clever he thought my husband was.

I had to leave with nothing. Goodbye Prada bag, Gucci heels, Chanel watch, Louis Vuitton belt, Dior sunglasses . . . and look out husband.

I got back on the train, so grateful for my phone and passport but couldn't speak. By the time I got back to the hotel, it had been a 15-hour round trip. Gary was worried as he had been unable to contact me. The kids were jumping all over the beds in the hotel room. Gary looked at me quizzically and asked me where all the shopping bags were. I said nothing, I just showed him the RACV card and sat down. He realised that he had packed the wrong card, he felt terrible and went straight to the minibar to get me a really strong drink.

It was such an extraordinary life lesson for me. Everyone has asked me if I was angry at my husband but that is not what I was feeling. I was so grateful to leave that city, for my freedom, for the country I live in, for the beautiful landscapes and for the safety that we have in Australia every day. I experienced so many emotions that day – nervousness, excitement, wonder, anticipation, impatience, fear, disbelief, relief, gratitude – it made me feel so alive. It was one of the most memorable days of my life as I really had no idea what was going to happen next and I absolutely loved it, even though I came home with nothing. I hope there are many more years ahead filled with adventure for me.

I hope if I make it to 99 years of age, I will still have a sense of adventure and excitement about the day ahead. I don't want to be 99, regretting the adventures I didn't take. Adventure is defined as excitement and a willingness to do new, unusual or risky things. It can involve travel, career, following your dreams, expressing your true feelings and love. We all have joys, hopes, fears, and longings that never go away, no matter how old we get.

A song close to my heart is Ronan Keating's 'I Hope You Dance'. The chorus goes: When you get the choice to sit it out or dance . . . I hope you dance.

And this is how I hope to always live my life.

I love this quote as well:

> You know, sometimes all you need is twenty seconds of insane courage. Just literally twenty seconds of just embarrassing bravery. And I promise you, something great will come of it.
>
> Benjamin Mee, *We Bought a Zoo*

Be courageous, live a life of adventure and not regret, no matter how old you are. Which brings me to my next chapter . . . While a life worth living includes adventure, the greatest adventure of all is love . . .

Chapter 4

Love and connection are the key to longevity

Love – the greatest adventure of all. The reckoning and yearning of the heart.

There are so many types of love. The love of a parent, a friend, a lover, a life partner and most importantly the love of self. The quest for love over our lifetime is certainly our greatest and most complicated.

In later chapters I will talk about how to improve your well-being and chances of living longer by exercising more or eating better, but did you know that maintaining meaningful, loving relationships plays a crucial role in health, happiness and longevity?

In the 1930s, Harvard University began the longest study on human happiness. For over 75 years, they did interviews, medical tests, and checked up on their subjects every two years to see how they were doing. Robert Waldinger is the fourth director of the study. In his TED talk, 'What makes a good life? Lessons from the longest study on happiness,' Waldinger says that while many young people tend to think that fame, fortune and hard work will bring them happiness, it's actually our social connections that are most important for our wellbeing.

The three major findings of the study are:

1. Social connections are really good for you, and loneliness kills. In the study, the people who were more socially connected to family, friends and community were happier, physically healthier and lived longer than people who were less connected.

2. The number of connections you have is not as important as the quality of your close relationships. People who valued quantity over quality when it came to relationships had poorer health and were less happy than those who had fewer, quality relationships.

3. Having high-quality social connections is not just important for your body, but it's also good for your mind. Waldinger said that subjects in the study with better social relationships had sharper memories than those in poor relationships. People in poorer relationships showed a steeper memory decline.

It is not just the strength of our relationships that predict longevity, however, but also the attitude with which we engage in those relationships that predicts a longer and healthier life. While we think we need to find someone to love us, research shows that some of the greatest benefits for longevity and wellbeing come not from receiving love but rather from giving love to others. An intriguing new study on loving-kindness meditation (LKM), a practice that involves generating love for others and is Buddhist in origin, shows that people who practise generating love on a regular basis have reduced cellular aging and telomere shortening. Telomeres are the caps on the ends of our chromosomes that protect them from damage and are an indicator of aging at the cellular level. Shorter telomeres are associated with higher incidences of disease and mortality.

It is the practice of making someone feel like they are needed, being connected, showing compassion and empathy that makes our lives so much more worth living. Compassion is the ability to show kindness, caring and a willingness to help others and it is proven that when you have high levels of compassion, not just for others but for yourself, aging slows down.

Are you the love of your life?

Self-love and acceptance is a very hot topic at the moment and for good reason.

When I was a young girl if you thought you were good at anything you were called 'up yourself' (I am not sure if that is only an Australian term) and that was the absolutely worst thing you could possibly be. There is a very big difference though between this and self-acceptance. Now we know how important it is to teach our kids self-acceptance and not to be too hard on themselves.

This is equally important for any woman my age. We are far too critical of ourselves and we need to stop it.

We also need to try to reckon with our uncontrollable hearts and to stop yearning for our completion through another. Love of self is so extraordinarily important because we shouldn't attach our sense of self-worth to something or someone else.

Having a strong sense of self and self-worth allows us to stay immune to criticism and not become reliant on the praise of others.

There is a fabulous new word that made it to the urban diction-ary in 2015:

Unfuckwithable – adj. – when you are a person who is truly at peace with yourself, and nothing anyone says or does bothers you, no negativity or drama can touch you.

This comes from a place of self-worth and self-love. Yep, self-love is the greatest middle finger of all time.

Vishen Lakhiani goes on to explain in his book *The Code of the Extraordinary Mind* that:

Extraordinary minds do not need to seek validation from outside opinions or through the attainment of goals. Instead they are truly at peace with themselves and the world around them. They live fearlessly – immune to criticism or praise and fuelled by their own inner happiness and self-love.

When we approach life from a perspective of self-love, we tend to prioritise our health more as well. Our reason 'why' we do what we do changes. We start to see things such as going to the gym or taking the time to eat in a healthy way as an act of self-love. We may previously have decided that we didn't have the time and that it wasn't a priority, but when our perspective around this changes, we make these things a habit and they even become enjoyable, as they are an expression of self-love. Self-love includes all of the things I talk about in later chapters such as maintaining a balanced diet, exercise, getting enough sleep and meditation and looking after your appearance.

When we increase our self-love and acceptance, we tend to make choices more often which are kind and loving to ourselves. You can never really meet your full potential until you truly learn to love yourself. It is important to note here that self-love is not narcissism. Narcissists believe they are better than others and won't acknowledge or take responsibility for their mistakes and flaws. They also seek enormous amounts of validation and recognition. Narcissists also lack empathy for others.

Self-love, on the other hand, isn't about showing off how great you are. People who love themselves in a healthy way know that they are flawed and make mistakes and they accept and care about themselves despite their imperfections. Self-love doesn't prevent you from caring about others; it simply means you can give yourself the same kindness that you give to others.

As we grow up, various situations, incidents and comments erode our sense of self. Human beings crave validation from other people as we are biologically hardwired to belong in a tribe. One of the greatest threats that can happen to us is being kicked out of the tribe as thousands of years ago, that meant being left to die. This is why what people think of us is so important and why negative feedback from others can have a detrimental effect on us psychologically.

It is extremely important to practise self-love. You can do this by:

- saying positive things to yourself
- forgiving yourself
- being assertive

- not letting others take advantage of you
- prioritising your health and wellbeing
- spending time around people who support you and build you up (and avoiding people who don't)
- asking for help
- letting go of grudges or anger that holds you back
- recognising your strengths
- valuing your feelings
- living in accordance with your values
- pursuing your interests and goals
- challenging yourself
- holding yourself accountable
- accepting your imperfections
- setting realistic expectations
- acknowledging your progress and effort.

> You yourself, as much as anybody in the entire universe, deserve your love and affection.
> Buddha

Just like Romeo and Juliet

When we have learned to love ourselves deeply, we have so much more love to share. Our relationships automatically improve as we operate from a greater place of love. Self-love affirms our identity, the life choices we make and allows for more happiness and deeper connections with others.

Romantic love is that supreme emotion that can affect everything we feel, think and do. That feeling that there is something larger than ourselves when we connect with the right person and a positive emotion runs through our brains and bodies all at once. It is an extraordinarily uplifting and powerful feeling. It's when we know that intimacy is not purely physical. It's the act of connecting with someone so deeply you can feel their soul.

As humans we have a deep desire to find real love and connection in life. To find a true union of love you need to be living in integrity with yourself and then approach your search with intention and authenticity. This is becoming harder and harder as dating apps can be based on all things that are superficial! Working out who you are, what your true values in life are, learning to love yourself and be honest in what you want for yourself is key. To find a soul partnership you will need to make sure you have healed all past hurts and done your own inner work so that you can be ready for your soul mate. Become your best self first.

I love Katherine Woodward Thomas' book *Calling in 'The One'*. Are you calling in the one, do you want to elevate the connection with the one you have or are you calling in the next one?

According to Thomas, the quest for 'the One' is difficult as there is a huge gap between wanting to find your ideal partner and being truly available . . . when he or she appears. You need to be prepared to let love into your life. You need to define your own identity, what you truly want and be committed to creating that future by letting go of all your past hurts.

I have always been a people-pleaser and ignored my own needs and I need to be accountable for the choices I have made because of this. Ignoring my needs and expectations means I am not being truly honest with myself or my partner.

The fulfillment of your vision and finding your soulmate is outside your old story, you are not a victim but accountable for what happened to you in the past and also for what you want to create moving forward. Who do you need to become and what character traits do you need to develop to attract 'the One' into your life? Thomas goes on to say that this psychological insight is only the beginning of the journey. You must then take massive action towards evolving yourself and becoming the person you need to be in order to bring 'the One' into your life. This is an extremely powerful message and very different from the romantic fairy tales on TV that I watched growing up.

Before I finish here, I should mention that self-love is important in every type of relationship, not just romantic love. Getting to know who we are and learning to love ourselves creates a solid foundation of self that we can bring to any relationship.

We are fortunate to live in a time when relationships can unfold at a pace that is right for us and take unique forms. Friendship, dating, open relationships, long-term relationships, long-distance relationships or committed relationships – we are free to choose the kind of relationships that we want.

Finding the relationship we want can come early or later in life. It may even happen again and again in one lifetime. There is no right or wrong for how to find a relationship nor is there a timeline that you have to follow. Follow your heart, listen to your inner voice, continue to become your own soulmate, and stay open to love. The journey of finding the right relationship begins with being in the right relationship with yourself.

Love really is the energy of life. While the heart's function is to pump blood around our bodies, it is also considered to be the place from which love starts and the place where love is received. It is no surprise then to learn that so much of longevity is tied to love. When your heart stops, life stops, so we could say that life begins and ends with the heart in more ways than one.

Chapter 5

The miracle of meditation

I have always wondered why some people are more vulnerable to life's ups and downs and others are more resilient. Why are some people more vulnerable to stress, depression, anxiety and fear while others seem to roll with the punches and get on with things?

Many people know that stress can shorten our life but did you know that stress can notably age your face and skin? Stress and anxiety can prematurely age our skin by:

- making our eyes appear darker and puffier
- deepening wrinkles
- weakening collagen levels (collagen is the structural protein)
- making skin drier
- encouraging skin inflammation.

So how do we take control of our stress levels? Before I start on how to combat stress, I will run through exactly what stress is and when it becomes bad for us.

Stress is your body's way of responding to any kind of demand or threat, whether it be real or imagined. When you feel threatened, the nervous system sends adrenaline and cortisol into the body and your heart pounds faster, your blood pressure rises and your breath quickens.

When working properly, stress can help you stay focused and energetic and help you rise to meet challenges. It can help keep you on your toes during a work presentation, sharpen your concentration in an exam or get that game winning shot. It is only good, however in short bursts.

If you become stressed frequently, as we all do because of today's demanding world, the overload on the nervous system can increase the risk of heart attack and stroke, speed up the aging process and leave you vulnerable to depression and anxiety.

You very often hear people saying they just want to live a stress-free life. I am right there with them, as I say this a lot myself. I think I say at least once a month that I am throwing it all in and moving to the magnificent Victorian countryside. However, in reality, there will always be times when stressful situations cannot be controlled. The only thing you can do is control your response to stress.

> Between stimulus and response there is a space. In that space is our power to choose our response. In our response lies our growth and our freedom.
> Viktor E Frankl

The most stressful thing that has ever happened to me was at Ringwood Hospital, Melbourne. My eldest son Luke, who was 25, had a cyst removed two weeks prior and we were waiting to see the doctor for the follow-up appointment. The doctor walked in and announced, with absolutely no bedside manner or warning, that it was cancer. We had not been at all prepared for this. Time stopped, everything went silent and seemed to be moving in slow motion. This couldn't be real. All I could do was wish that it was me and not him. How could I take this away from him so that he wouldn't have to go through it?

The worst thing about a cancer diagnosis is the unknown. You have to wait a couple of weeks for test results to come in so that you know exactly the type and the stage of cancer and if it is treatable. Luke and I would go on the internet together, all hours of the night trying to work it out. I would try to be strong in front of Luke, telling him that it would work out but it felt as many describe, like drowning, suffocating and not being able to get back up to the surface.

The only thing you can do at this point is to try to control your mind and emotions, and work through it one step at a time. This is where meditation became my saviour. I will always be in awe of the brave way that Luke handled this from the first moment of his diagnosis, through to learning the cancer stage.

The day finally came when we would be told Luke's prognosis. Everyone in the waiting-room honestly had white hair. You could hear a pin drop, nobody uttered a word. How could this be happening to my son in his mid 20s? We waited for 30 minutes, it felt like days.

Finally we saw the oncologist, and I could feel I was holding my breath, trying to remain calm. We learnt that he was going to be okay and the overwhelming feeling of gratitude made me fall apart in the doctor's office. I am not sure I could have made it through this time in my life without meditation. It kept me in the space of doing what we had to and helped to manage the over-whelming anxiety of what may happen in the future.

Not all stress is caused by external factors. Stress can also be internal or self-generated, when you worry excessively about something that may or may not happen or have irrational, pess-imistic thoughts about life. What causes stress depends, at least in part, on your perception of it. Something that's stressful to you may not faze someone else, they may even enjoy it. While some of us are terrified of getting up in front of people to perform or speak, others love the spotlight. Where one person thrives under pressure and performs best under a tight deadline, another will shut down when work demands escalate.

Our brains are constantly being shaped by the forces around us and most of the time we have little control over this, but we can start taking more responsibility for our brains. It is possible to take responsibility for our own states of mind – and to change them for the better. We now know that there are obvious connections between our psychological wellbeing and our systematic health. This is where the practice of mindfulness and meditation comes in. Changes in the brain can happen quickly and if we nourish our mind for a small time every day we can truly change our world.

Meditation is shown to thicken the pre-frontal cortex. This brain center manages higher order brain function, like increased awareness, concentration and decision-making. Changes in the brain show, with meditation, higher-order functions become stronger, while lower-order brain activities decrease.

Have you ever seen a Buddhist monk looking stressed? I love the Dalai Lama – he has the most beautiful face and smile. I am not a Buddhist, but he fascinates me. You can see he is so full of the best human qualities, kindness and compassion and he is so happy. He has lived an amazing life full of happiness and joy. Can I have some of that, please? Buddhist monks meditate, every day.

Meditation has certainly changed my life and is now a crucial part of my daily routine. It is essentially familiarising yourself with the present moment. If you decide to live in the present moment, let go of the past and are not afraid of what may happen tomorrow you can experience dramatic improvements in your life. Meditation is about being aware of your thoughts, watching them come and go without judgement. It is the progressive quieting of the mind until it reaches the source of thought.

Meditation will help you to stop overthinking things. Overthinking causes you to live in the past or the future instead of the present. So many people are controlled by their overthinking minds and this can cause a great amount of mental suffering, stress and anxiety. It will also teach you to focus on the task you are engaged in. A research paper came out of Harvard that showed our minds are distracted 47% of the time and that mind-wandering is a direct cause of unhappiness.

It is amazing the benefits you will see when you learn to separate yourself from your mind through meditation and stop over-thinking. The psychological and physiological benefits include:

- feeling less threatened
- being less reactive
- feeling more rested
- being more creative and open to possibilities
- sleeping better
- blood pressure lowers
- immune system is boosted
- generally, your overall health improves
- the aging process is slowed.

Why wouldn't anyone want to meditate given its benefits? The mind is our most precious and valuable resource and we use it to experience every single moment of our life. We depend on our mind to be focused and perform at our very best, yet we don't take the time to take care of it. This can be done in as little as 15 minutes per day. The great news is that there are some amazing apps available for your phone that will teach you how to meditate and make it extremely easy and enjoyable for you to practise it every day. Or you can google meditations – one of my favorites is *Gratefulness* by Deepak Chopra.

I make sure that I meditate first thing in the morning and then in the afternoon to make sure I am on track with what I am trying to achieve that day. I look forward to it because it makes me feel good. After 15 minutes I feel refreshed and focused and ready to take on the next challenge for the day. It makes me feel stronger and more centered. It makes me more productive as it stops me from being distracted. As with many things you will really see the benefits after you have practised it consistently. It might take a few weeks to get into the habit, but it will be worth it.

While many think that this is a time waster and that their to-do list is far more important, waking 15 minutes earlier to do this simple process can be transformative. It is probably more important to do it when you are feeling the most rushed and the list of tasks is exceptionally daunting. Pausing for meditation makes a huge difference in getting you in the right frame of mind to tackle the day ahead.

Not only does meditation reduce my stress levels and stop me from overthinking, it also allows me to take control of my emotions. Being able to control your emotions is a very powerful thing. Our minds are easily manipulated and mental toughness is about emotional control. When you learn to control your emotions, you control your choices. When you can control your choices, you take control of your life.

> . . . everyone has ability. It always comes down to mind games.
> Whoever is more mentally strong, wins.
> Muhammed Ali

If practised consistently, meditation will not only reduce your stress levels, it will make you mentally strong. So if you want to achieve a big goal, start meditating. It will help you consciously create a life you love as you will take the time to get clear as to what you want out of your life.

The other great thing about meditation is that as you start to plug into a source of internal fulfillment, this allows you to become a giver, not a taker. When you find internal fulfillment you find that you want to help others. It can create extraordinary life shifts. You start asking: what can I give, contribute or offer? I bet your favorite person is internally fulfilled and when you talk to them, it is like you are the only person in the room. They have time to listen and are generous.

I started my journey with guided mediation apps which are mindfulness meditations. They are directed meditations that deal with your stress right now. As you practise this and you no longer need to be guided, you can access a deeper healing state that has been proven to stop sickness, stress and slow aging.

Ask for the life that you want when you are meditating and watch how it unfolds itself to you.

Section 2

Nike got it wrong – you need to *'Just do it every day'*

You have to be mentally ready to make changes for the betterment of your future self and once you are, it all comes down to one thing and that's the nitty gritty of getting it done. Repeated action, habit. This is why there are so many books on creating great habits.

This section talks about the way to get from where you are to where you want to be. The you on the other side. There is only one way and that is to do something.

You have to commit to continually do the things that will make you that younger, healthier version of yourself. Not just once or twice but for the rest of your life. Make a promise to yourself and keep it, your ageless self depends on it.

Chapter 6

The compound effect

Nike were missing two words when they made their slogan. Instead of 'Just do it' it should have been 'Just do it . . . every day'.

I am a total personal development addict. I can't count the number of conferences I have been to or the number of books I have read. I totally believe that the books you read today will shape the person you become in the future. I have been to a couple of PD conferences in the US and at one of them, I came across a presenter who had me from the moment he started talking. His name is Darren Hardy and he has written a number of books, but the one that has had the most profound effect on me is called *The Compound Effect*.

The compound effect is where small, seemingly insignificant steps taken consistently over time will create a radical difference. That's it. Be the turtle and you will always win. You don't have to be the smartest, the fastest or the strongest – you have to be the most consistent. Most people can't sustain what needs to be done over a longer period of time, however this is what will ultimately lead to success. Small choices, but the right ones, consistently.

Modern marketing has brainwashed us into thinking that we can achieve everything instantly, but this is not the case. The problem is that we expect instantaneous results without the required effort. I have definitely been guilty of this. You know how it is, after one day of eating correctly, you get on the scales the next morning and you haven't lost the expected couple of kilos . . . damn it! Or you exercised and still no movement on the scale. Well, here is the thing, it has taken you . . . (fill in the blank) number of years to get where you are now, so it's not going to change in a day, a week or even a month. Instead, it's going to take you making responsible decisions about your health and wellbeing, consistently, for the rest of your life.

Here are some examples of the compound effect.

Let's start with wine, which is a recurring theme in this book as it is definitely a weakness of mine. I love a great chardonnay and can drink two glasses of it very quickly. I decided to drink red instead, a really yummy pinot noir. As I drink red more slowly, I now only have one glass of wine in the evening. Let's do the maths over a period of a year. You will save approximately 200 calories a day × 365 days = 73,000 calories. As a general rule of thumb, you need to be in an energy deficit of around 7,000 calories (29,400 kilojoules) to lose one kilogram of fat. That's a loss of 10kg over the course of the year.

Let's say that you choose to forgo the muffin you have every day with your morning coffee. A muffin has about 350 calories.

Let's do the maths on this one – 350 × 365 = 127,750 or approximately 18kg. Seriously, is that muffin really worth it?

And if you have also taken up running four times a week for 30 minutes (read Chapter 14) that's an average of 400 calories per run. 400 × 4 × 52 = 83,200. That's about 12kg a year.

There you go, some running, one less glass of wine and one less muffin daily over a 12-month period and you are cooking with gas! The problem here is that even though the results are massive over time, the small steps you are taking in the moment don't feel like they are significant enough. So you have the extra glass of wine or have that muffin or stop running.

Stay the course . . . be committed to yourself. Even if you were to start by taking an extra 500 steps a day, that's an extra 182,000 steps a year, which is an extra 146km.

Small steps every day towards your goal are the only way to move forward. It is the same in all aspects of your life. It took me seven years of part-time study to complete my Accounting degree while I was raising my son and working full-time. But I got there in the end. All you have to do is stay the course and remain consistent with small achievable goals. This principle will apply to many facets of your life where it is the constant repetition of an action that provides the benefit over a long period of time. Examples include resistance training, meditation, studying, your skin care routine, saving money, building a database of clients or building a respected brand name, just to mention a few. The best thing about the compound effect is that it is predictable and measurable. As long as you take the small steps every day you can radically improve your life. Isn't that better than feeling like you have to be superhuman over a small timeframe only to fail?

The snowball effect

Once you understand the benefits of the compound effect, it has a profound influence on the way you think. When you see the benefits and significant impact that one small change consistently can have it starts to have a snowball effect, as the confidence it builds leads you to taking more positive steps forward. The snowball effect is a long-term process that starts from an initial state of minor differences and builds upon itself, just like when a snowball rolling down a hill becomes larger and larger. A snowball can turn into an avalanche if it gathers enough force along the way. Imagine how your life would be if the same force was propelling your mental and physical actions forward. The compound effect turns into a snowball effect that creates extraordinary positive momentum in your life.

An example of this is how taking the small consistent step of exercising daily creates momentum and has a positive effect on the brain. Did you know that exercise makes you smarter?

Here's how:

Exercise produces endorphins, which improves the prioritising functions of the brain. After exercise, it is much easier to block out distractions and better concentrate on the task at hand.

Your brain remembers more when your body is active because the endorphins, also known as nature's mood elevator, have been shown to improve memory. Exercise also releases serotonin, which improves mood and alleviates symptoms of depression. It improves your brain in the short term by raising your focus for two to three hours afterwards. The more you move, the more energised you will feel. Regular physical activity improves your muscle strength and boosts your endurance, giving you the energy you need to think more clearly, come up with new ideas and be more creative. Working out boosts growth hormones that promote new nerve cells. It releases other brain chemicals as well that help cognition such as dopamine.

You thought you were only getting fitter but you're getting smarter as well!

The compound effect teaches us that to reach our goals, overcome obstacles and become the best version of ourselves, this will not happen by taking shortcuts. There really is no other way than to take action, so the discipline of small steps taken consistently will reap great rewards.

Small, smart choices, consistently over time, WILL change your life. What are you going to promise yourself that you will do every day, non-negotiable, that will create your longer, happier, healthier, more ageless life?

Chapter 7

The danger of neglect

In order to stay young both physically and mentally we must make sure that we don't neglect ourselves.

> What's simple to do is also simple not to do.
>
> Jim Rohn

Exercise is simple, so is eating well and meditating. These things are also very simple not to do. The secret to living a longer, happier ageless life is not difficult, yet we still don't do what we should to look after ourselves. In fact, the primary reason most people are not doing as well as they could be can be summed up in a single word: neglect.

Neglect is like an infection. Left unchecked, it will spread throughout our entire system and eventually lead to a complete breakdown of a potentially joy-filled life.

Not doing the things you know you should do will cause you to feel guilty and guilt reduces your self-confidence. Then a negative snowball effect starts to happen. As your self-confidence reduces, so does the level of your activity. And as your activity reduces, you don't achieve your goals. When you don't achieve your goals, your attitude starts to worsen and as your attitude turns from positive to negative, your self-confidence diminishes even more. This is when you start beating yourself up, comparing yourself to others and feeling like you are not good enough. And it all started with you neglecting to take action.

So why do you neglect yourself? Why do you hold yourself back from looking after the most important person in your life? For some reason, many of us think that making the time to put ourself first is somehow self-centred. In a lot of cases, it's because you are feeling so stressed running around looking after everybody else, kids, partners, friends, parents, that it is really hard to make the time. Taking care of your mind and body isn't selfish, and you shouldn't feel guilty about setting some time aside. It's incredibly important to maintain a healthy lifestyle because it reduces stress, increases confidence and gives you a more positive outlook on life.

For some, a reason you neglect yourself is by letting work take over your life. Whatever your work demands, you need to make sure you take steps to stop it from taking over your life and look after your wellbeing. Unrealistic deadlines and ever-increasing demands can be overwhelming. The stress this creates can be very damaging to the mind and the body. It is very easy for neglect to happen when we are juggling work and family. But you must prioritise yourself and make time or the consequences of the accumulated stress due to lack of self-care can not only rob you of the life you deserve but can cause illness and be life-threatening.

Self-care really is not selfish, but for some of us, we have been brought up to believe that it is. So many people that I talk to, especially in my generation, think this for many reasons. They seem to have an inner voice telling them that it is uncaring if they look after themselves first. They think that sacrificing their own needs for someone else's makes them a good person and that self-care is something that you only do occasionally as a reward. They just feel flat out guilty for doing anything for themselves.

Taking care of yourself is actually the opposite of being selfish. Looking after yourself is how you combat stress and build resilience. It builds up your energy and strength which in the long run will help you to look after your loved ones. A bit like putting on the oxygen mask in a plane first before you can help anyone else.

So how do you look after yourself? I have tried to summarise all the ways you can look after yourself in this book. It will result in a much happier, healthier, younger you. However, in order to really know where you should start in your journey of turning around self-neglect, you will need to listen to your own inner voice. In order to do this, you will need to stop worrying about everyone else because while you are trying to analyse everyone else's needs, you won't be able to work out your own.

I have made a list here of some things to consider as you read through the book. Listen to your gut instinct, it will tell you where you need to start first. You can't do it all at once, so just start with the thing that you think might have the most impact for you at this stage in your life. As you start to take action, the reverse will happen to neglecting yourself, it will build your self-confidence and create positive momentum.

- drinking water
- being present in the moment and not being distracted
- actively practising gratefulness
- practising mindfulness and meditation
- resistance training
- 30 min cardio
- smiling
- learning when you need to say no to someone
- being aware that you are overthinking
- stopping any negative self-talk
- having fun
- looking after your hair, teeth, skin
- general check-up with your doctor
- treating yourself after achieving a goal
- recognising your achievements
- planning something that excites you
- spending time with people that make you feel good about yourself
- not worrying about what others think
- getting enough sleep
- being true to yourself, not who others want you to be
- eating nutritious foods
- reducing sugar
- limiting social media time
- avoiding negative fear-mongering media

- personal development
- keeping in mind your passion and your why
- being gentle and patient with yourself
- forgiving yourself
- truly connecting with others
- prioritising your own needs
- being aware of the opportunities around you
- embracing uncertainty and adventure.

It doesn't matter what is going on in my life – my philosophy is that I will do one thing today and every day that I will thank myself for tomorrow. What are the everyday small things you think you could include in your daily life? It's amazing how the small things make huge changes.

Chapter 8

Be the tortoise

Winning is not determined by how fast you start.
Winning is determined by how long you last.
Darren Hardy

I am literally the tortoise. I keep plodding along until I get to where I want to be no matter how long it takes. Slow and steady doesn't only win the race, it achieves all your life's dreams and goals. The tortoise is a great way to picture how to be resilient. Pop back into that protective shell for a while if you need to and then pop back out again and keep plodding along with a clear picture in your mind of where you want to be. One foot after the other. It works. You need to create an environment which enforces great habits and enables you to keep moving forward even in the face of adversity.

The things I discuss in later chapters to age in a new way will not work unless you incorporate them into your life and make them a habit. There is an enormous amount of literature on how to create good habits and there is a reason for that. Aristotle nailed it.

We are what we repeatedly do. Excellence, then, is not an act, but a habit.
Aristotle

Are you living on autopilot and letting your habits run your life? This is great if you have healthy habits but a disaster if you are eating junk food every day. The ultimate purpose of a habit is to solve the problems of life with as little energy and effort as possible because once your habits become automatic you stop paying attention to what you are doing. But are your habits working for you or against you?

We cannot rely on motivation. It is a fickle thing that comes and goes. You will not be motivated every day as motivation fluctuates with your emotions. So don't feel bad on the days you are not motivated. Understand that this is normal and that you need to create habits and discipline that will see you through a bad day or a rough patch.

The silver bullet, the magic pill doesn't exist. But the life hack does. It is creating consistently good habits. You have to do the work and you are the only one that can make it happen. If you start eliminating bad habits and creating great ones, you will see the changes happen. The smallest changes to your daily routines can drastically change the outcomes in your life.

So how do you replace bad habits with good habits? What is going to stop you from falling back into bad habits without thinking? Where do you even start? Rather than focusing on what you want to achieve you need to focus on who you want to become. This is key. How you identify yourself will determine what actions you take. If something is an important part of your identity you will automatically create the habits required to maintain that identity. Your identity is directly connected to your highest values, your core self, your why. This is where you will find the greatest motivation that will bring about consistent change and good habits.

Success is not something you pursue. Success is something you attract by the person you become. If you want to have more you must become more.

Jim Rohn

Who do you need to become to achieve what you want and what is most important to you? For habits to change, you need to change. If you really want to make big improvements in your life you have to know who you want to become and why. If your why isn't strong enough, you just won't stick at it.

When you have established your why, how do you go about eliminating bad habits and installing good ones? What has worked for me is changing them one at a time. Remember some of our habits have been part of our lives for decades, so we need to be consciously aware of these automatic behaviours. My health is one of my core values so drinking two litres of water a day is a simple but life-changing habit I have had to force myself to do. The only way I could make myself do it was to fill a two-litre water bottle every day first thing in the morning and stick it right next to my computer. Some days I wouldn't get through it but that was okay. I would always congratulate myself for the water I had managed to drink. I am a coffee in the morning and a wine in the evening type of girl and adding the water habit into my life helped me to reduce my coffee and wine intake. Remember it doesn't have to be perfect, but it has to be an improvement, a continuous improvement.

The reason the water bottle worked is because habits are initiated by a cue. It is extremely important to create environments with the right cues. You need to be aware of what cues and environments are creating your negative habits and which people cause you to make the wrong choices and try to avoid them where possible.

When choosing a habit to start with it is important to understand keystone habits. Keystone habits are small changes or habits that people introduce into their routines that unintentionally carry over into other aspects of their lives. For example, people who exercise regularly tend to eat healthier, sleep better and are more likely to be productive at work. Keystone habits make it easier to start other good habits, build your confidence and make positive behaviours addictive.

I have a keystone habit that impacts all the other areas of my life. Every night before I go to bed, I spend five minutes making a list of what needs to be done the next day. Then I go through the list and look at what is important to me and achieves my big goals and what is urgent but serves the agenda of others. It also includes any running around for the kids and chores. I then cross off anything that is a plain waste of time or can be done another day and then look at anything else where I could possibly enlist the help of friends or family members. Next, I delegate any work items that my staff could do. With the items left, I prioritise them in order of importance rather than urgency. This is so empowering because I sleep well without worrying about what I need to do the next day. I get out of bed and know exactly what I am going to do first. And most importantly of all, I am creating daily habits that are helping me work towards my goals.

Remember to be patient with yourself. The human brain has evolved to prioritise immediate gratification over delayed rewards and when you are aware of that you can start to make changes. Creating new habits will take time though. Especially if the habits you are changing are 30 or 40 years old. There will be times when you give up, so remember that this is normal and get back into the routine of the good habit.

I saw one of the most amazing speakers I have ever seen when I was in the States. Jocko Willink was a Navy Seal whose military service included combat in the war in Iraq and he achieved the rank of Lieutenant Commander. Now if you want to learn how to achieve great habits and discipline, Jocko is an incredible thought leader and role model. He has written a book called *Discipline Equals Freedom*. What resonated the most with me about what he said was that at the end of the day you can't control other people, you can't make them who you want them to be; the only person you can control is you. This is extremely liberating.

So focus on making yourself who you want to be. With the right habits you can discipline your body and free your mind. You can become faster, stronger, smarter, more humble and have less ego. Get after it and you will become the person you want to be.

One small decision at a time.

Chapter 9

The captivation of confidence

My life philosophy has been that I will always do one thing today that I will thank myself for tomorrow and it has definitely worked for me. Just one thing in my crazy day or crazy life and it has meant that I have never lost myself completely to the overwhelming world we now live in. I have kept an element of control.

It is the smallest things that count, but you must take action. How you look and talk and walk all relate to the level of self-confidence you are currently feeling. Walking tall and feeling great about yourself can instantly make you look years younger. There is something so sexy and attractive and young about a confident person – they seem to have a particular aura that you want to be around. We all know someone that is particularly attractive simply because of the way they carry themselves. The person they are. The way they smile. They are magnetic.

Confident people seem to carry the fountain of youth around with them. Confident people are happy with who they are as they take a sense of pride and pleasure from their accomplishments rather than from what other people think. Confident people don't pass judgement on others as they don't need to bring other people down to feel good. Confident people listen actively and pay attention to others as they don't feel they have anything to prove. Confident people see opportunities and take them, fear doesn't hold them back.

So how do we become more self-confident? Self-confidence is a skill that can be and needs to be learned and developed. It is not something, as many may think, that we are born with.

Inaction breeds doubt and fear. Taking action builds confidence and courage.
Dale Carnegie

We all struggle with self-confidence and so many of us believe that we aren't good enough. Confidence is the willingness to try something new, because when you try and you take action you start to believe that you can become that person. Action builds experience – you don't have to be perfect, you have to start. Experience builds confidence.

Dr Ivan Joseph has presented an amazing TED Talk on self-confidence. His definition of self-confidence is 'the ability to believe in yourself so that you can accomplish any task no matter the odds, no matter the adversity, no matter the difficulty.' He believes that it is a skill that needs to be trained, and the easiest and only way to build self-confidence is through repetition. Taking an action over and over again. We cannot be confident unless the skill or action we are taking is not novel to us. Sometimes the problem with repetition is that we stop after the first failure and therefore stop the repetition. We have to remain persistent with our actions.

My middle son Ben is a great example about repetition and confidence. He has played basketball since he was four years old and after many years of driven, hard work and finishing year 12, he was invited to a four-year college in California to try out for a basketball scholarship. Ben is a point guard who is six feet with shoes on. There was no certainty here. It was a week of visiting the campus, tryouts and training sessions. For weeks before we went, Ben practised his three-point shot for hours. Long, repetitive hard work.

I travelled to California with Ben. When we arrived, it was not only extremely exciting but extraordinarily nerve-racking (for me anyway). We went to watch the games, and I felt like I was on the set of an American movie. College games are a big deal in the States, many of the games are televised. Halfway through the first quarter of one of the games we were watching, the commentator came over to us in the stands and asked if Ben would throw a half-court shot for the halftime entertainment. I was so nervous because the head coach would be watching. At half-time they announced him on to the court as the prospect from Australia. My heart was in my mouth. Ben picked up the ball and put the half-court shot straight through . . . swish! He had the ability but also the skill of self-confidence from hours and hours of repetitive work which allowed him to perform under pressure.

The story continues. We had been there for four days, and Ben had been to all the training sessions. The head coach came over to me and said that Ben was doing very well but he wouldn't be making any decisions until the final training session the next day and that he would have a meeting with us in his office directly after that. I didn't sleep that night and the next morning, we were at the court early, waiting for the coaches. They came in and behind them was an All-American basketball player who had graduated from this College and was about to start playing professional basketball.

Again, my heart was pounding out of control but Ben was calm. This guy was a giant and African Americans have such extraordinarily athletic physiques. The training started with ball bouncing drills. I sat and watched and was unable to move. After some more regular drills it was time for a shooting competition between Ben and the All-American. They would shoot from nine designated spots around the key and three-point line and when your shot went though you would move to the next spot. First one around five times wins. It started and I watched, frozen. Ben was calm and moved further and further ahead of his opposition and the coaches watched with a look of amusement on their faces. He won, the All-American had to get down and give the coach 20 push-ups. The coaches put down the basketballs they were holding and clapped Ben. I started breathing normally again and couldn't wipe the smile off my face. My six-foot son felt 10 feet tall.

I knew that Ben had the ability but I was so in awe of how he stayed calm and showed the confidence to perform under pressure. I was a mess all the way through. That confidence comes from hours of repetitive action.

The next part of confidence building also involves repetition. It is the repetitive thoughts we have, the things we repeat over and over in our head. Thoughts do not just influence our actions, they determine them. The most important words we say all day are the words we say to ourselves. Our self-talk will determine our actions, which will in turn determine our self-confidence.

Self-confidence has two major components. The first is that you are certain of your abilities, which is achieved through action and repetition. The second is the belief that you are valuable, worthwhile and capable, which can be achieved through the repetitive thoughts you impress on your subconscious. These two things combined will enable you to act confidently and courageously. The only thing separating you from your grandest vision in life is action and courage.

There are many books on affirmations and visualisation. A popular response to these books is that you can't think you are going to achieve a goal and it will magically happen. Of course not, but there is a definite science behind it and without it you won't be able to achieve anything.

Some of the best personal development books written focus on the power of your thoughts, such as:
- *Think and Grow Rich* – Napoleon Hill
- *The Power of your Subconscious Mind* – Dr Joseph Murphy
- *As a Man Thinketh* – James Allen

Put as simply as possible, you will automatically do and create what your mind is subconsciously thinking about. The subconscious mind believes what the conscious mind repeatedly tells it. The subconscious mind goes about creating whatever is most greatly impressed upon it. This is therefore why you need to be very careful about the thoughts you are repeating over and over about yourself in your head.

When words, whether they are true or false, positive or negative, are embedded in the subconscious, your mind goes to work with all its faculties and energies to materialise them in real life. So if you have a goal and you bury it deep in your subconscious mind through repetitive thoughts and having a clear picture of what you want to achieve, your subconscious mind will go about taking the action required to create that. And as you start to take action you will develop self-confidence.

To become the confident person you would like to be, you need to create a mental picture of your newly conceived self and continually hold onto it.

What is the one thing that you will take action on today that you will thank yourself for tomorrow and that will help build your confidence? Whatever it is, just do it and keep doing it . . . every day.

Section 3

You have to embrace the basics first

We tend to associate food with weight, but it is so much more than that. The basics for a long and healthy life start with exactly what we put in our mouths. The purpose of food is nutrition. Some of us view it as an evil when it really is the 100% source of our health and longevity. Changing how you think about food can change everything. If we think about food as the way to support the billions of cells in our bodies and the antioxidants as a way to fight free radicals (including cancer cells) and also as a way to slow all the aging traits, it is easier to make better choices. It has taken me a long time but I now view highly processed foods as 'food-like substances' which have no nutrition and that is how I stopped eating them. It is easy to love beautiful, fresh food and making a few simple changes can be the difference to a much longer life.

Chapter 10

You are NOT on a diet

Losing weight, or being the correct weight, is one of the most transformative things you can do. It can take decades off your physical appearance. There are literally thousands of diet books out there all claiming to have the silver bullet, the secret way for instant weight loss, but if it took you 40 or 50 years to get to the weight you are today, you are not going to instantly change that with a magic diet in a couple of weeks. We know this to be true; it is common sense.

We need to have a healthy diet and thought process around food for the rest of our lives. We must have generally good eating habits that include eating fruits and vegetables, avoiding junk food and unhealthy snacks, avoiding binge or emotional eating, drinking enough water and just making sure that our bodies are receiving the basic nutrition they need. This is for the rest of your life, not a restricted diet for a short period of time.

Lasting transformation is not about restrictive rules. It's not about being told you can do this or you can't do that. It's about changing your psychology and how you think about food. If you want to get different results, then you have to do different things. Your health is 100% determined by making sure that your body gets enough of what it needs. Physical fitness will only make you healthier if you have the correct nutrition.

What if you started changing the way you talk about food and instead of saying 'I am on a diet' you started saying, 'I am making sure that my body receives all the nutrition it needs'? Health is more than wealth. A strong and healthy body translates to a fuller, happier life. So while switching to a healthier diet is not easy, the benefits are definitely worth it.

To change your health, wellbeing and longevity you need to change your relationship with food. As human beings we have certain nutritional requirements and needs such as vitamins and minerals, proteins, amino acids and fibres.

Your body doesn't want to be overweight, it wants to be healthy and strong. When you eat processed foods and sugars however, your body becomes full of toxins and it can't function the way it should and that's when you start to build up fat cells. It is important to understand that weight and health are not separate issues. It is unhealthy to be overweight. Lots of very overweight people are malnourished. A high calorie diet is generally not high in vitamins and minerals.

So it is not just about calories in and calories out. We need to avoid foods that are high in toxins and choose foods that are full of nutrients. To do this we need to eat food in a state that is not highly processed. All highly processed foods contain sugar.

Sugar

When I was growing up, the way to eat was low fat. What we didn't know back then was that nearly everything advertised as low fat was high in sugar and carbohydrates. Sugar is now one of the biggest health issues of our generation. Low-fat diets full of processed sugar will only make you gain weight, undermine all your body's nutritional needs and make you age prematurely. Major health studies from the World Health Organization have issued statements that we must dramatically cut our sugar intake. There are several reasons:

1. Sugar makes you fat. Your body will always burn sugar first before it burns fat. Excess sugar, which the pancreas turns into insulin in the bloodstream, prevents ketosis from occurring, which is how your body burns fat. Ketosis is a process that happens when your body doesn't have enough carbohydrates to burn for energy. Instead, it burns fat and makes things called ketones, which it can use for fuel.

2. It is now proven that eating too much sugar and being over-weight drastically increases your risk of illnesses such as certain cancers, Alzheimer's, heart disease and diabetes. Sugar wears out your pancreas and kidneys as they try to deal with a substance they shouldn't have which causes them to fail – this is essentially diabetes. When you eat excess sugar, the extra insulin in your bloodstream can affect the arteries all over your body. It causes their walls to get inflamed, grow thicker than normal and more stiff, and this stresses your heart and damages it over time. This can lead to heart disease such as

heart failure, heart attacks and strokes. Sugar has also been implicated in Alzheimer's disease. Some scientists even refer to Alzheimer's as type 3 diabetes. This is because of the difficulty for people with Alzheimer's as their brains seem to have trouble in breaking down glucose, the brain's main source of energy.

3. Chances are that you already know eating too much sugar isn't good for you. But did you know that it is addictive? Sugar makes you crave more sugar. Eating sugar gives your brain a huge surge of a feel-good chemical called dopamine, so when your blood sugar drops your body craves more. The excess sugar in your blood also gives you a quick burst of energy which is fleeting and leaves you feeling more tired than you were before and once again craving more sugar. The multi-billion-dollar food manufacturers know this – they add it to foods unnecessarily without any regard for our health to make us buy more food so they can continue to increase their profit margins.

4. Sugar causes inflammation throughout our body, and as a side effect, this makes your skin age faster. The inflammation causes damage to collagen and elastin in your skin, the protein fibres that keep your skin firm and youthful. The result? Wrinkles and saggy skin.

5. Sugar can increase cellular aging. Telomeres are structures found at the end of chromosomes, which are the molecules that hold part or all of your genetic information. Telomeres act as protective caps, preventing chromosomes from deteriorating or fusing together. As you grow older, telomeres naturally

shorten, which causes cells to age and malfunction. Although the shortening of telomeres is a normal part of aging, unhealthy lifestyle choices can speed up the process. Consuming high amounts of sugar has been shown to accelerate telomere shortening, which increases cellular aging.

6. Studies have shown spikes in sugar intake suppress your immune system. When your immune system is compromised, you are more likely to get sick. If you eat a lot of foods and beverages high in sugar or refined carbohydrates, which the body processes as sugar, you may be reducing your body's ability to ward off disease.

We all know of white refined sugar but sugar is also found in many other places. Fruit juices are full of sugar. So are white breads, pasta and rice, packaged cakes, biscuits and muffins. Many foods labelled as low-fat including yoghurts, salad dressings, breakfast cereals and cereal bars contain hidden sugar. Drinking soft drinks is like pouring sugar down your throat. Our bodies have not adapted to eating these highly processed foods. A processed food is one that has been altered to extend its shelf life and looks nothing like food in its natural state. The less a food has been tampered with, the better it is for your health. These foods will not only make you fat but they will keep you malnourished as they hold no nutritional value. They also contain additives such as flavourings and colourings that can be harmful. We need to eat carbohydrates in their most natural state which is fruit and vegetables.

So you can see that you really need to give up sugar in all its forms if you want to live a long, healthy life. It comes named in many different ways on the side of packaging so don't be tricked. All words ending in 'ose' are sugar. Artificial sweeteners are full of toxic chemicals so you will really need to steer clear of them as well.

The thought of giving up sugar can be quite overwhelming to some. Sweet is the first taste that humans prefer from birth. I will have a couple of squares of low-sugar dark chocolate so I don't feel like I am being completely denied. If you feel the need to have something with sugar in it, try to keep it small – less than 150 calories.

Alcohol

I love a great glass of wine.

Red wine has been studied for many years and did you know that most people who live past 100 enjoy a glass of red wine every night? Red wine is abundant in resveratrol. Resveratrol is a plant compound that acts like an antioxidant. The top food sources include red wine, grapes, some berries and peanuts.

Red wine can promote longevity because of its relaxation effects. Long-term population studies have linked moderate red wine drinking to a longer life. Research also suggests that you strengthen the effect of resveratrol by pairing it with a nutrient-dense diet of vegetables and fish (similar to the Mediterranean diet).

There have been numerous studies on resveratrol that show it has properties that can promote blood flow to the brain to sharpen the mind, may help reduce pressure on the artery walls and lower blood pressure, combat inflammation on the body, reduce insulin resistance and has been linked with a lower risk of developing heart disease.

Despite all of the above reasons, too much alcohol is not good for us. Alcohol is full of sugar and contains phytoestrogen which promotes fat storage and decreases muscle growth. The body also has to process alcohol before it can process any other food you have consumed. Alcohol therefore causes weight gain because it stops your body from burning fat. It is high in calories, it can make you feel hungry and it can lead to poor food choices.

The key here is moderation; too much can be destructive to your health, making you fat, raising your blood pressure and your risk of developing several kinds of cancer. Avoiding it completely might hold you back from some of the benefits that moderate drinkers enjoy, like lower incidence of cardiovascular disease and type-2 diabetes and increasing longevity.

I generally have a glass of red wine most days. Although I love white wine, I try to avoid it because I tend to drink it far too quickly which generally means I am reaching for another glass.

So what should I eat?

You can tell by looking at a food whether it is over-processed as it will not look like something in its natural state. For example, an avocado looks exactly the same as it does when it is on the tree. The food doesn't look like it has been tampered with. There are no added toxic preservatives to make it last in your cupboard for six months or artificial flavours to make it taste a certain way. There is not a long ingredient list full of things you can't pronounce and sugar isn't one of the major ingredients.

How do you feel after you have eaten the food? Usually after eating highly processed food you will feel bloated and tired. Take notice of this and remember how you felt as it may make you make a better choice next time. A salad with olive oil, high quality protein and some beautiful herbs will make you feel full and alive!

This is a general list of the foods I include in my diet: I have incorporated them into a sample seven-day menu at the end of this chapter. You will see from the recipes I like to keep things simple.

Proteins

Proteins are made up of chemical 'building blocks' called amino acids. Your body uses amino acids to build and repair muscles and bones and to make hormones and enzymes. They can also be used as an energy source. Every cell in the human body contains protein. The basic structure of protein is a chain of amino acids. You need protein in your diet to help your body repair cells and make new ones.

Study after study has shown that people who have a high protein diet:

- lose fat faster
- gain more muscle
- burn more calories

- experience less hunger
- have stronger bones
- have better moods.

I am not a vegetarian and so I have not included non-meat proteins, however I do not feel that you need to eat meat every single day. Apologies to my vegan friends. Proteins to include daily:

- salmon
- tuna (fresh steaks, not tinned)
- any white fish such as John Dory and barramundi
- beef
- chicken
- duck
- lamb
- turkey
- eggs.

Vegetables are king

Leafy green vegetables are an important part of a healthy diet. They're packed with vitamins, minerals and fibre but low in calories. Eating a diet rich in leafy greens can offer numerous health benefits including reduced risk of obesity, heart disease, high blood pressure and mental decline. The vitamin K contents of dark green leafy vegetables provide a number of health benefits including: protecting bones from osteoporosis and helping to prevent against inflammatory diseases. Because of their high content of antioxidants, green leafy vegetables may be one of the best cancer-preventing foods. Ultimately, they will help you live longer! Vegetables to eat include:

- asparagus
- avocado
- broccoli
- Brussel sprouts
- cucumber
- green beans
- kale
- mushrooms
- onions
- green pepper
- rocket
- spinach
- sweet potatoes
- tomatoes
- zucchini.

Fats

Growing up it was drummed into me that fat would make me fat. This is not the case, and oh how I wish I had learned this sooner. Sugar gives us premature wrinkles and makes us sick and hungry. The right kind of fats, however, can make us look younger and reduce hunger cravings. The right kinds of fats come from nuts, seeds, oils, meat, fish and seafood. These kinds of fats slow the rate at which sugar hits your bloodstream, which will mean you won't feel hungry. Good fats also help us to absorb vitamins and minerals more efficiently. Include these good fats in your cooking:

- avocado oil
- macadamia nut oil
- extra virgin olive oil
- coconut oil
- nuts
- oily fish
- seeds.

Dairy

I tend not to have dairy as it makes me feel bloated and uncomfortable. I prefer almond milk and I will also have small amounts of high protein yoghurt. Cheese is full of saturated fat, and while I love it, I will only have small amounts. Many people find that they are lactose intolerant and also that excessive milk consumption has a long association with increased respiratory tract mucus production, asthma and general inflammation.

Nuts and seeds

Mounting evidence suggests that eating nuts and seeds daily can lower your risk of diabetes and heart disease and may even lengthen your life. Nuts are highly nutritious and loaded with antioxidants, good fats and fibre. They are high in calories so you need to limit the amount you eat. They are great for a quick snack or to put in a salad to make it really yummy. Try these nuts and seeds:

- sunflower seeds
- pumpkin seeds
- sesame seeds
- macadamias
- cashews
- almonds (not roasted)
- walnuts
- pecans.

Fruit

I love fruit but eat it in limited quantities because of its high sugar content. I generally eat it at breakfast. Although fruit is packed with goodness, the majority of the fresh food we eat should be vegetables. Add these fruits to your meals:

- apples
- pears
- watermelon
- rockmelon
- blueberries (especially high in antioxidants)
- strawberries
- nectarines
- peaches
- oranges.

Flavourings

One of the most important things you can do for your health is to take out the added flavourings in food full of chemicals and sugars. We all have that friend that puts sugary tomato sauce on everything! The items listed below will bring out the natural flavours in food rather than covering them up:

- Extra virgin olive oil
- sesame oil
- sugar-free and gluten-free soy sauce
- lemon
- lime
- dill
- parsley
- rosemary
- thyme
- basil
- chillies
- garlic
- tumeric (also an anti-inflammatory)
- mustards.

So now you know what to eat and why, how do you incorporate it into your daily lifestyle permanently? Be organised, prepared and keep it simple when cooking. You will learn to love simple fresh food. It is so much more tasty and satisfying than over-processed sugary foods.

I haven't eaten a McDonald's burger for 30 years as not only are they toxic, I think they taste disgusting.

I have provided a week of simple recipes below for you that I absolutely love, but if you are going to incorporate this into your life permanently you are going to have to look for recipes that you love. I have found the easiest way to do this is to google 'keto' recipes which are generally inclusive of protein and vegetables. Avoid the recipes that are high in cheese and dairy products, instead you need to increase the level of high quality vegetables and proteins you are eating. If you then need to add carbohydrates (I always do this after strength training to grow muscle) I add things like roasted pumpkin to a meal or oats to my breakfast or protein smoothie. You will learn over time what you like and what works for you.

Planning and being prepared is crucial. If you don't have the fresh food you should be eating in the fridge, you are setting yourself up to fail. You will end up eating some overly processed piece of rubbish in your pantry that has no nutritional value and is full of carbohydrates and sugar. The best way to start planning is to choose what meals you will be eating for the week ahead. When you know what you will be eating it is then easier to plan for the ingredients you will need to have in the fridge. I have a saved list online with the local supermarket and have it delivered which saves me heaps of time.

A quick word on eating out and incorporating this into your new life plan. You don't have to stop going to a restaurant, you have to be aware of what you are ordering. Melbourne is known for its fabulous restaurants and one of my favourite things to do is to eat out. Avoid ordering things like bread, potatoes, pasta and rice, it fills you up anyway and stops you from enjoying the really delicious food you could be eating. My absolute favourite food is a great Teppanyaki. You can see the freshness of the food the chef is preparing right in front of you.

Fall in love with food that is good for you and make it part of your life. Learn how to stop eating food that has no nutritional value and is reducing your life span and making you fat. In the next chapter I will talk about the psychological and behavioural changes you may need to consider to help you along.

A sample weekly eating plan

Breakfast	Lunch	Dinner
Egg stack with 2 poached eggs on top of ham, and pan-fried spring onion, tomato and mushrooms	Chicken salad with bacon, spinach, avocado, cherry tomatoes, and a dressing of olive oil, apple cider vinegar and Dijon mustard	Spiralised zucchini spaghetti with pine nuts, pancetta, spinach leaves, feta, olive oil, salt and pepper
Protein shake in Vitamix or Nutri bullet with whey protein, water or almond milk, blueberries and a handful of macadamias or walnuts	Speedy portable lunch – mix together some cooked chicken with sweetcorn, cucumber and mayonnaise	Pan fried eye fillet with Dijon mustard and roasted asparagus

Breakfast	Lunch	Dinner
2-egg omelette with turkey breast, mushrooms and spring onions	Chicken fillet, roasted pumpkin, red pepper, spinach, zucchini, cauliflower, walnuts, olive oil, salt and pepper	Roasted salmon fillet, spring onion, asparagus, broccolini, cherry tomatoes, soy sauce, sesame oil, sesame seeds
Gluten-free oats with almond milk, Pro Yo yoghurt and strawberries	Bolognaise meat sauce with zucchini noodles or broccolini	Caprese chicken – Pan fry chicken fillet on both sides in olive oil, top with Italian seasoning, bocconcini, avocado, tomato, add lid and cook through, top with balsamic glaze
Toasted Burgen bread (wholemeal and seed) with avocado and feta cheese	Frittata – red onion, red pepper, zuchini, goats cheese, eggs	Stir fried Asian vegetables, ready-chopped (from fruit and veggie section at supermarket) with salmon and teriyaki sauce (low-sugar from health food shop)
2-egg omelette with ham, red pepper and red onion	Pan fried bacon, mushroom, cherry tomatoes, small broccoli florets, olive oil, cracked pepper	Stir-fried chicken thigh fillets with mushrooms, beans, onions, garlic, paprika, olive oil
Scrambled eggs with smoked salmon and spinach	Salad of crabmeat, zucchini, avocado, rocket, pine nuts, chilli (optional) with dressing of olive oil, lime juice, mustard and mint	Slow cooked lamb shanks with stir-fried green beans, red pepper and cauliflower rice

Chapter 11

Did you really enjoy that donut?

Is your answer to the question above: yes, absolutely loved it and I want five more; or is it: not as much as I thought I would? In many cases we know we are going to feel bad after eating the food we think we crave but we eat it anyway. Why do we do that? Did you know that the first few bites of a food taste better than the next few bites, and after a large amount, we may have very little taste experience left at all? It is your thought process around food that will ultimately change your behaviour and your life. If we all know what to do, then why don't we do it? Why are we making the food choices that we do? This is the real answer to lasting change.

So how do you make long-term lasting improvements to the way you eat because you know this will increase the quality of your life now as well as your longevity? You know that a diet is a temporary change to the way you eat in order to achieve a short-term goal and does not work in the long run as it is not sustainable. You know that looking for instant results with the latest diet craze on instagram is crazy, right? You know that diets are a waste of time because you are looking for the quick fix and haven't changed your basic eating habits. You know that dieting isn't healthy and that choosing to limit what you eat in a specific way until you lose a certain amount of weight won't work because you will just go back to your old eating habits. So why keep doing it?

Diets fail people. It is really important therefore to stop beating yourself up, let go of the past and be excited about the healthy changes you are going to make for yourself, now and permanently into the future. You deserve to be healthy and happy. Right now, you can decide that you will make different choices consistently, not just for a couple of weeks but for the rest of your life, which will allow you to live longer.

It all starts with your mind and the story you are telling yourself about food. Any change in your body happens in your mind first and that is where you must start to make lasting change.

The way you start to do this is by listening to the conversations you have with yourself around food. What reasons do you give yourself to eat toxic foods that harm your health? Perhaps there are reasons like: I worked out really hard today so I deserve it. How are you convincing yourself that it is okay or that you need to eat something you know you shouldn't? Do you associate foods with certain feelings? Is it the taste of the food driving you to eat it or is it an emotional experience you had in the past that you are trying to recreate that you attach to that food? Do you finish your plate because you were told as a child you had to because there were so many starving children in the world?

Did you know that if you tell your subconscious mind something enough times it starts to believe it and your conscious mind then starts to behave accordingly? Your subconscious mind is subjective. It does not think or reason independently; it merely obeys the commands it receives from your conscious mind. Start telling yourself that you are a healthy person who hates disgusting donuts because they make you sick, fat and age prematurely. Tell yourself that for two weeks straight and then try to eat a donut and see if you enjoy it. Stop telling yourself that one won't hurt because you are lying to yourself and until you work out why you're lying to yourself, the nutritional value of your food won't change.

This is why it is so important to understand why we really get hungry so that we can start to make real changes to the way we eat.

According to Eric Edmeades, who is the founder of WILDFIT, there are six primary hungers that drive your eating decisions. When you begin to understand what those six hungers are, when they come up you know what to do about them and sometimes, that's not eating.

1. Thirst hunger

Historically most of the food we ate as cavepeople had a high-water content. Cavepeople didn't have bottles to carry water around with them, so when they became dehydrated and thirsty the first thing they would look for was fruit and vegetables, or food that is high in water. If you are dehydrated, your body may be craving water-based foods (not a bag of chips which will make you thirstier). Drinking six to eight glasses of water a day will stop this type of hunger and the motivation to eat will go away.

2. Emotional hunger

Food is often associated with past emotions. When we are feeling emotionally susceptible, we try to fix this with food. You need to notice how you are using food to satisfy an emotional need and to be aware that this is happening. Do you have particular foods that you go to when you are feeling really down? How do you think the food is going to make you feel? Did it make you feel that way? If you recognise that this is happening, you will be able to deal with these sorts of emotions without having to reach for food.

3. Low blood sugar hunger

This is that feeling at about three o'clock in the afternoon when your energy levels are starting to fade. This is because your body is using mainly sugar as a food source which creates highs and lows in energy levels. When blood sugar levels dip below a certain range, you may experience certain symptoms like lack of energy, headache, shakiness or irritability. This means that a less-than-normal level of sugar is available in the bloodstream. If sugar has been the main source of energy for our body's cells, and the cells cannot get the energy they need, you may feel hungry, unable to concentrate, or just feel overall irritable. The minute you start to feel low blood sugar you immediately want to eat something with carbs in it and so the cycle continues.

Your body can burn sugar or it can burn fat. When your body switches over to burning fat, the state of ketosis, these symptoms will stop. Your body needs to learn how to become good at this and to do it efficiently and effectively. When you realise that you can change your metabolism and that your body can receive a steady form of energy, this will eliminate a huge need for snacking and eating dysfunctionally.

4. Empty stomach hunger

We associate the feeling of an empty stomach with hunger but the two are very separate things. Our stomachs are designed to be expandable and shrink again, however in the Western world we never allow our stomachs to be empty. It is actually a good thing to empty our stomachs, as this allows our intestines to clean themselves. When we realise that an empty stomach is simply a feeling and not an indication of hunger, we can really start to make some changes.

5. Variety hunger

The reason for this is that we need a variety of foods to satisfy our huge nutritional requirements. Sometimes you may need to change things up a bit in order to feel satisfied. This does not mean a variety in junk food! Are we getting a variety of all the right healthy foods? We are so overwhelmed by the variety of non-food-like substances which are highly overprocessed and offer no nutritional value on the supermarket shelves that this can make it even more confusing and overwhelming.

6. Nutritional hunger

This is the only type of genuine hunger, the rest of them are illusory. If you are running low on a particular vitamin or mineral your body will seek out this food. Remember there is absolutely no nutritional value in donuts (or the like) and this is how food companies make money out of you. They produce high-calorie low-nutritional food to stimulate you to eat more than you need of these types of foods.

When you start to fill your body with the nutrition it needs it will stop feeling hungry. Plant food, proteins and water will reduce your nutritional hunger dramatically. Understanding this can start real change in your relationship with food. This is called conscious consumption. We want to make sure that we are eating real foods full of nutrients and not something that is chemicals and sugar in a plastic wrapper. In order to do this, we need to be aware of the choices we are making and why.

So how are you talking to yourself about food? Do you know which type of hunger is making you eat? Is it real or a perceived hunger? How are you talking yourself into eating food that is bad for you? It is only when you start to realise why you are eating the wrong foods that you can make lasting changes.

Reducing stress and eating consciously can help us make better food choices as we will start to opt for more real foods rather than products pretending to be foods. We will start to ask: is this food that has come from the earth and provides nutritional value or is it something that has been adapted and mutated? These extremely important questions could add decades to your life as well as make you look decades younger.

It is important to mention here that stress will not only lead you to bad food choices but that it can also make you fat. When you are in a constant state of stress because of a relentlessly busy lifestyle your body releases the hormones cortisol and adrenaline, which are fat-storing hormones, into the bloodstream. The foods we turn to normally in this situation such as sugar, coffee and alcohol continue to flood the bloodstream with toxic substances that are actually stress inducing. Nutritional foods can help counteract stress so you are far better off to choose foods such as nuts, berries, green leafy vegetables and avocados.

Eating with awareness helps us to eat the right type and amount of food, avoid overeating and helps us to identify how certain foods make us feel. Understanding how food makes us feel helps us to make better choices and feel good about our lifestyle. The next time you find yourself reaching for a donut (or the like), ask yourself why you are about to eat it and maybe you will make a different choice.

Chapter 12

The foundation of anti-aging – water and sleep

Living a healthy life sometimes is hard and challenging. We all face obstacles in our life and never seem to have enough time to truly take care of ourselves. The reason I have included sleep and water together in the same chapter is because they are very simple things you can improve on that can make a huge difference mentally, emotionally and physically. They will not take a lot of your time, just some simple tweaks. Proper amounts of water and sleep are key components to our mental and physical health, our wellbeing and longevity.

We are always told to drink eight glasses of water a day, but how many of us actually do that?

I am going to explain here the reasons why, so next time you find yourself not drinking enough water you can just remind yourself why it is so important. When you truly know why you need to do something you are far more likely to do it, as knowing why drives our behaviour.

Your skin is an organ. In fact, it's the largest organ in your body, and it's mostly made up of water. Without water, your skin can't function at its best. If your skin doesn't get enough water, not only will it become dry, tight and flaky, but it will also become even more prone to aging.

While there are so many reasons to drink water from a biological perspective, one of the keys to anti-aging is water. Our body is approximately 60% water so therefore the key to staying young is hydration. Drinking enough water means the water stays where it needs to be, inside the cells. Water plays an important role in the wrinkles and pores of your skin. Without the correct water intake, your skin will seem duller, dry and actually prone to wrinkling. If you are properly hydrated, your skin will become plump and the elasticity will improve. This will help keep your skin looking young, and you will be less likely to develop wrinkles. Hyaluronic acid, which I will talk about in later chapters, works by allowing your skin cells to hold onto more water, which creates a plump, dewy complexion that looks younger.

Water helps you from the inside out. For your skin's sake, it's one of the easiest and best beauty treatments you can do. Not only will it reduce wrinkles, it will improve the complexion and reduce puffiness. It does this by helping your digestive system flush out toxins from the body and by increasing the blood flow to the skin, which will improve your complexion for healthy, glowing wrinkle-free skin.

The other really awesome thing that water can do for your appearance and overall health is help you lose weight. It does this in a number of ways. It is a natural appetite suppressant. It takes up space in the stomach and as you feel more full, you will eat less. Sometimes we think we are hungry when we are actually thirsty so if you have a glass of water first it can stop you from snacking. A lack of water and dehydration causes our body to retain toxins. When waste builds up in the body you start to feel bloated and tired, so staying hydrated is a good way to avoid retaining waste, which may add a few extra pounds. Drinking enough water is also essential for burning off stored fat. The process of metabolising fat is called lipolysis and this cannot be done efficiently without water.

There are so many reasons for our health to drink water, including having a great workout. For our focus on anti-aging, it keeps your skin clear and plump and will slow down the development of wrinkles and it is essential for metabolising fat. The majority of us don't drink nearly enough water so go and fill a glass up and get it into you. As most Australians aren't drinking enough water there are even water apps now that have easy to use water trackers and motivating reminders.

Sleep

Let's talk about sleep now. Beauty sleep is a real thing. Some of us think we can burn the candle at both ends and live on a limited amount of sleep but you pay for it. Poor sleep results in premature aging because it is when we are asleep that the growth hormone is released.

Dr Jacob Teitelbaum, author of *From Fatigued to Fantastic* says the following:

Also known as the 'Fountain of Youth' hormone, optimizing growth hormone keeps us young. It keeps our muscles toned, and our skin at its full thickness. Think of it as a healthy facelift for your entire body, including face, breasts and abdominals. Sleep also plays a critical role in our production of two key hormones that regulate appetite and weight gain. These are leptin and ghrelin. Numerous studies have shown that inadequate sleep results in an average 6½ pound weight gain and a 30 to 55 percent higher risk of obesity.

I think we all know that getting a healthy night's sleep isn't just a way to keep the wrinkles away, it will also make you healthier. It rejuvenates your mind and body, it increases energy levels and gives you more vitality. Sleep highly influences your cognitive performance and is also emotionally healing. It shapes every facet of our lives as well as our sense of wellbeing. Sleep is vital for recovery and repair for all the functions of our body both physical and mental.

So if you are struggling with sleep, as many of us are, what do you do?

We need at a minimum approximately seven hours of sleep a night. Sleep is regulated by two hormones, melatonin and cortisol. Cortisol helps you wake up in the morning and melatonin levels rise at night to make you sleepy. So we need to protect our melatonin levels in the evening. This can be done in a number of ways.

The first and one of the most powerful ways to improve sleep is keeping regular hours. It is referred to as our body's circadian rhythm, our sleep wake cycle or our body clock. Getting up at the same time every day anchors our circadian rhythms and gives our bodies the cue that is time for us to be awake. We become increasingly awake and then as the day passes increasingly tired and if we disrupt this pattern it is harder for us to get to sleep at night.

Try to go to bed at the same time and wake at the same time, as this can be very effective sleep training no matter what your age. It might be tempting to watch one more episode of whatever you are binging on Netflix but your sleep schedule is too important as a regular sleep pattern can also improve the quality of your sleep. Don't check your emails or procrastinate – go to bed and have a routine. I know it's boring, but extremely important if you are struggling with sleep.

Another one of the most powerful things you can do to aid sleep is exercise. The more regularly you exercise the better you will sleep. It uses up energy and regulates our metabolism, our hormones and circadian rhythms. Exercise will help you fall asleep faster and stay asleep longer. Moderate aerobic exercise, which can be as simple as 30 minutes of walking, increases the amount of time you spend in deep sleep. Deep sleep is the stage where your body restores and replenishes itself.

Light-emitting screens are a problem. Our bodies and our delicate circadian rhythms were built to respond to daylight, not the around the clock availability of electricity and illuminations of televisions, phones, computers and the like. When exposed to more light our bodies produce less melatonin and therefore we find it harder to go to sleep. You may have heard about blue light being a particular problem. Light is made up of the seven colours of the rainbow and in the daytime we require blue light to wake us up and make us alert. Natural sunlight or bright light during the day helps keep your circadian rhythm healthy. This improves daytime energy, as well as night-time sleep quality and duration.

However, the screens we look at in the evenings emit this blue light. Harvard researchers have found that blue light suppressed melatonin production, shifting our circadian rhythms by three hours and reducing the quality of sleep as well. So a good idea is to turn down the light emitted from your devices as evening approaches and to spend time in more dimly lit rooms.

This brings me to creating the right environment for sleep. Room temperature can make or break your sleep quality. The best room temperature for sleeping is 18–20 degrees Celsius, which allows you to fall asleep and stay asleep. Body and bedroom temperature can profoundly affect sleep quality as you may have experienced during the summer. Keep the bedroom dark and quiet. Get some block-out blinds if you need to and remove any artificial lighting. If you live in a particularly noisy area you could invest in earplugs or headphones and download a white noise app. I love an open window as well (probably because I am a terrible claustrophobic) as this reduces carbon dioxide which improves sleep quality.

We all know that caffeine is a stimulant and should be avoided in the afternoon as it will prolong the time it takes you to fall asleep. But what about alcohol? Although alcohol helps us to relax and fall asleep quickly it actually reduces melatonin production and leads to disrupted sleep patterns. Drinking alcohol heavily or too close to bedtime affects your sleep cycle and quality. The first half of your night's sleep may be okay but the second half will be very disrupted as your body needs to metabolise and get rid of all the toxins you have taken in.

I mention meditation many times throughout this book and it can be just as helpful to induce sleep. When you meditate, a variety of physiological changes occur. These changes initiate sleep by influencing specific processes in your body. It increases melatonin, the sleep hormone and increases serotonin, the precursor to melatonin. It reduces the heart rate, decreases blood pressure and activates parts of the brain that control sleep. As a result, meditation can promote sleep by initiating these changes. Whatever type of meditation you do will reduce stress and anxiety, which are two of the most common causes of insomnia.

What happens when you wake up in the middle of the night and can't go back to sleep? This is so frustrating and then you find that you fall into a deep sleep just before the alarm goes off! This usually happens because something is playing on your mind and really worrying your subconscious. Maybe you spent the day with an anxious person who has passed their anxiety on to you. Things seem so much worse at 3am. Best thing to do is to get up and read a book, refocus the mind, don't stay in bed wide awake for hours. And the next day, avoid that anxious person and their toxic energy that they are passing on to you.

Vitamin D, calcium and magnesium

Vitamin D is a great supplement as it decreases your risk of osteoporosis, some cancers and heart disease, but did you know it is also a great way to improve your sleep? It is proven that people with low levels of vitamin D in their blood take longer to fall asleep and find it harder to stay asleep. This is because vitamin D is important for the efficient transporting of calcium around the body. Calcium is directly related to our cycles of sleep. Researchers have found that calcium levels in the body are higher during some of the deepest levels of sleep, such as the rapid eye movement (REM) phase, and that disturbances in sleep are related to a calcium deficiency.

Poor sleep is also common symptom of magnesium deficiency. People with low magnesium often experience restless sleep, waking frequently during the night. Maintaining healthy magnesium levels often leads to deeper, more sound sleep. Magnesium is also good for the reduction of stress and anxiety.

Chapter 13

Fasting is so much more than losing weight

None of us are ever perfect all of the time! There will be times when you have over-indulged and you need to drop some kgs. I have found that if I need to lose weight, fasting is the only thing that works for me and it works quickly. I was the same weight for 15 years after my last son was born and I just couldn't drop those last 5kgs. Then I tried fasting and they disappeared.

As a weight loss approach fasting has been around in various forms for ages, but was highly popularised in 2012 by BBC broadcast journalist Dr Michael Mosley's TV documentary *Eat, Fast and Live Longer* and book *The Fast Diet*.

There are other reasons why fasting is such a popular topic at the moment. There are studies now showing that going into a fasting state does more than help us burn calories and lose weight. Dr Valter Longo is a revered professor of biochemistry and director at the University of Southern California's Longevity Institute and has studied fasting diets for many years. Professor Longo says there is a range of benefits you can get from fasting and that going without food can propel some genes to function better in repairing our body. Fasting not only helps with weight loss but also in the reduction of age-related diseases including Alzheimer's and dementia as it allows the repair genes to work more effectively and gives your pancreas a rest.

Numerous studies have seen tremendous health benefits that may occur during or following fasting. Some noteworthy benefits include:

- decrease in blood sugar levels and reduction of insulin resistance
- decrease of inflammation markers
- lower blood pressure, triglycerides and cholesterol levels, and therefore improved cardiovascular health
- improved brain function, increase in nerve cell synthesis and protection against neurodegenerative conditions
- delayed aging and increased longevity
- increase in levels of human growth hormone (HGH), an important protein hormone that plays a role in growth, metabolism, weight loss and muscle strength.

The truth is, our ancestors didn't have access to food like we do now. During times of scarcity, they would have to rely on fat stores for energy. They would fast.

So what exactly is fasting? The medical dictionary defines it as 'the voluntarily not eating of food for varying lengths of time. Fasting is used as a medical therapy for many conditions. It is also a spiritual practice in many religions.' It then goes on to say

'Fasting can be used for nearly every chronic condition, including allergies, anxiety, arthritis, asthma, depression, diabetes, head-aches, heart disease, high cholesterol, digestive disorders, mental illness, and obesity. Fasting is an effective and safe weight loss method.' Fasting is not starvation, but rather the body's burning of stored energy. Starvation occurs when the body no longer has any stored energy and begins using essential tissues such as organs for an energy source.

There are many reasons to make fasting a part of your life. From a medical standpoint, many diseases are caused from being overweight. Excess weight can raise your blood pressure, lead to arthritis, disrupt sleep, cause back pain and liver disease. Type 2 diabetes, which is closely related to excess body fat, is the number one cause of blindness, kidney disease and amputations.

Fasting regulates your hormone levels – it's more than a diet as it resets your body's internal controls, allowing you to burn the right amount of energy to keep you alive.

Avoid fasting if you have specific caloric needs. Individuals who are underweight, struggling with weight gain, under 18 years of age, pregnant or breastfeeding should not attempt fasting, as they need sufficient calories on a daily basis for proper development. Of course, if you have any underlying medical conditions you would need to talk to your doctor before you started any sort of fasting.

Where do you start?

Here are some of the popular ways to do intermittent fasting and the best way to start is to look at which one you could manage the best and fit into your lifestyle. I tend to do the 16:8 version as this is the one I find easiest. You can drink water, coffee and other zero-calorie beverages during the fast, which can help reduce feelings of hunger. It's very important to eat healthy foods within the eating window. It won't work of course if you eat highly processed and sugar laden foods or an excessive number of calories. Rather than referring to this as a diet you could refer to it as a pattern of eating to reduce your food intake and increase the use of burning fat for energy. When in a fasting state, the meals you eat will depend on the method you choose.

16:8 method

The 16:8 version involves fasting every day for 16 hours and restricting your daily eating window to 8 hours. Within the eating window, you can fit in two or three meals. Doing this method of fasting can actually be as simple as not eating anything after dinner and skipping breakfast, which is why I prefer it as I am not a breakfast eater.

For example, if you finish your last meal at 8pm and don't eat until noon the next day, you're technically fasting for 16 hours. For people who get hungry in the morning and like to eat breakfast, this method may be hard to get used to at first. However, many breakfast skippers instinctively eat this way. Others opt to eat between 9am and 5pm, which allows plenty of time for a healthy breakfast, a normal lunch around noon and an early dinner around 4pm before starting your fast.

The 5:2 method

The 5:2 version is eating normally 5 days of the week while restricting your calorie intake to 500–600 calories for 2 days of the week. This way of fasting is also called the Fast Diet and was popularised by British author Dr Michael Mosley.

On the fasting days, it's recommended that women eat 500 calories and men 600. For example, you might eat normally every day of the week except Tuesdays and Thursdays. For those two days, you eat two small meals of 250 calories each for women and 300 calories each for men.

Eat Stop Eat method

Eat Stop Eat involves a 24-hour fast once or twice per week. This method was popularised by fitness expert Brad Pilon and has been quite popular for a few years.

By fasting from dinner one day to dinner the next day, this amounts to a full 24-hour fast. You can also fast from breakfast to breakfast or lunch to lunch as the end result is the same.

It's really important to keep hydrated during this time and that you have a diet high in nutrition during the eating periods. The potential downside of this method is that a full 24-hour fast may be fairly difficult for many people. However, you don't need to go all in right away. It's fine to start with 14–16 hours, then build up from there.

The Warrior method

The Warrior method of fasting was popularised by fitness expert Ori Hofmekler. It involves eating small amounts of raw fruits and vegetables during the day and eating one big meal at night. Basically, you fast all day and feast at night within a four-hour eating window. The Warrior Diet was one of the first popular diets to include a form of intermittent fasting. This is a great one if you want to include vitamising vegetables during the day in the nutribullet and then eat protein and veggies at night.

Some tricks of the trade . . .

People tend to assume that hunger will increase during fasting, however it tends to decrease. During fasting your body switches fuel sources. Instead of relying on blood glucose, which is derived from food for energy, your body begins burning body fat, which is stored food energy.

This is called the state of ketosis. The time it takes to go into ketosis depends on the type of fasting you are doing, however once you begin ketosis your body has an enormous amount of calories it can tap into to use for energy.

The best way to start fasting is to start slow because you don't need to follow a structured intermittent fasting plan to reap some of its benefits. You can start by simply skipping meals from time to time, such as when you don't feel hungry or are too busy to cook and eat. It's a myth that people need to eat every few hours or they will hit starvation mode or lose muscle. As discussed above, our bodies are well equipped to handle long periods without food, let alone missing one or two meals from time to time. So if you're really not hungry one day, skip breakfast and eat a healthy lunch and dinner. Or, if you're travelling somewhere and can't find anything you want to eat, do a short fast. Skipping one or two meals when you feel inclined to do so is the easiest way to start intermittent fasting. Once you have started doing this you can build up to a longer, more structured method of fasting.

Stop snacking! You don't need to eat eight times a day and while you are doing this, you are always thinking about food, what you need to eat and when you need to eat it. Once you have become used to skipping the occasional meal and you have stopped snacking you can then reduce from three meals a day to two and you are on your way . . .

To finish, I will quickly cover fasted cardio.

Exercise while fasting makes your body burn a greater percentage of fat for fuel. If we run or walk fasted, we tap into our fat stores as a fuel source sooner, so we're exercising more on oxidised fat versus glycogen or carbohydrates. People who ran on a treadmill in a fasted state burned 20% more fat than those who didn't in a study published in the *British Journal of Nutrition*, and people who consistently trained in a fasted state over the course of six weeks showed more endurance improvements than those who ate before working out.

I like to run in a fasted state. Afterwards I feel great. It is not a highly intense workout though, which isn't recommended when you are fasted.

Fasting is not something that should be done when you are trying to build muscle. To lose weight, you need to burn more calories than you take in. You need to have a net calorie deficit. To build muscle, you need to eat more calories than you burn. You need to have a net calorie surplus of nutritional foods.

Section 4

After nutrition, exercise is everything

When I was growing up, exercise was something you did to stay thin. It was all about Jane Fonda and Richard Simmons jumping up and down on our TV screens burning calories. I wish I had known then what I know now because I would have included strength training as well as cardio in my exercise routine for the last 35 years.

Exercise really is the best defense and repair strategy that we have to counter different drivers of aging. As people age, they lose muscle mass and strength, a condition known as sarcopenia which is a natural cause of aging. This can be reversed however through resistance training. It is one of the best ways to help slow aging yet there are so many women my age who shy away from it. If you seriously want to slow the aging process, you will need to do a combination of cardio and strength training. It can be really fun and simple. Acquiring more muscle mass, no matter what your body type, is the foundation of a strong, anti-aging body.

Chapter 14

Cardio is better than Zoloft

A big statement, I know, but I have tried both. Firstly, let me say that I am not a doctor so definitely don't stop any medication you have been prescribed. There was a time in my life that I really needed help to get through a very painful time as I was not coping. Zoloft, a prescribed anti-depressant, did this – it helped me get to the other side for which I will be forever grateful. However, it also made me feel nothing – I felt numb and had no emotions and I didn't like that at all. Increasing my heart rate with cardio has had a profound effect on my mental as well as my physical wellbeing. Increasing your heart rate with cardio releases chemicals like endorphins and serotonin that improve your mood. It also pumps blood to the brain, which can help you to think more clearly.

I bet you think you can't run. Unless you have a medical reason not to, I am here to tell you that you can. I love to run. Mind you, I hated it when I first started but now it is one of the things I look forward to most in my day.

Only 30 minutes of running (or cardio such as cycling) can have huge benefits on your short-term and long-term health. I started out by walking and over the course of a couple of months found that running really wasn't as hard as I thought it would be. I will talk about how to build up to a 5km run but first let's talk about the why.

Don't get me wrong, when it's cold and I feel tired I think maybe I will skip my run today, but once you have started you catch the runner's high. Just 10 minutes of aerobic exercise releases a large amount of mood boosting endorphins. The benefits aren't only in the moment either: regular running has long-term effects on your mental health by decreasing stress and anxiety and improving energy levels.

The other thing that running for 15–30 minutes will do for you is kickstart your metabolism and burn some serious fat. You have got to love that! During a short run your body will use fat as its primary power source rather than carbohydrates. And here is a cool fact, once a workout is over and you're back in your daily routine, your body's metabolism will continue to be increased even when at complete rest. This is called excess post-exercise oxygen consumption, or EPOC. This can last from 15 minutes to 24 hours after your run.

So you are feeling good, boosting your metabolism and guess what else you are doing? Burning calories! You will burn between 200 and 500 calories in half an hour, which is an awesome way to lose weight or a guilt-free way to enjoy something you wouldn't have been able to otherwise without paying a price for your indulgence. My weaknesses are all things starting with CH, such as champagne, cheese, chocolate, chardonnay – so it would be one of these. (It just so happens that Chris Hemsworth is also a CH but I digress . . .)

Another good thing about only running for 30 minutes is that you will be at much lower risk of injury. This means it is a habit that you can continue.

Guess what else happens? Studies have shown that the increased fitness level you achieve from regular short runs can add years to your life expectancy. There are so many reasons for this – it will help regulate and lower blood sugar, strengthen the immune system, lower blood pressure, improve circulation, increase memory function, improve cholesterol levels, lower stress hormones. Basically, it will give you an all-round better quality of life.

When you start running regularly for 30 minutes you will also see your sleep improve significantly. You will fall asleep faster and spend more time in deep sleep. Sleep heals your body from the abuse of the day, fuels it up to tackle the next day and fortifies your organs to fight against future stress and disease.

You will look better and feel stronger. Running three to four times a week will show more defined muscle as the kilograms drop off the scale. Your skin will also start to look clearer and healthier due to the improved circulation.

Let's summarise those benefits:

- catch a runner's high
- boost your metabolism
- burn those calories
- lower risk of injury

- increase life expectancy
- improve sleep
- look better and feel stronger.

Read this when you don't feel like putting those runners on. Worth investing half an hour four times a week? Absa-bloody-lutely . . .

Tricks of the trade

Unless it's the weekend and I can slot a run in a bit later, I run first thing. If you get out of bed and exercise early you will own the day instead of the day owning you. Put your running gear next to the bed the night before and then as soon as your alarm goes off, get up and put it on. Another trick, if you are having trouble getting out of bed, is to put the alarm out of reach so you have to get out of bed to turn it off.

You have to invest in excellent runners otherwise you will injure yourself and will have to stop before you even get started. For the ladies, you must invest in a great bra otherwise you'll end up with a very sore back and shoulders. I wear a light waterproof jacket that I can take off halfway through the run when I warm up – or put back on when it's raining. Because I live in Melbourne, I never know what the weather is going to be. Next investment are airpods or something similar. Download a music app: I love Spotify. Now you are ready!

Drink a couple of glasses of water before you start so your circulatory system is working at its best. Make sure that your shoulders are back and you have good posture as this will make it easier to breathe. Breathe deeply into your stomach and try to keep a relaxed pose. I found when I first started that my knees were hurting. It was because my feet weren't hitting the ground properly and I was overcompensating. Go to the physio and get this sorted if this or something like it happens to you. It is 100% worth it. After all, the quality and longevity of your life depends on it.

How to build up to 5km

If you haven't run before you are not going to run 5km on your first day. You will need to build up to it over time. Remember that this is a habit you want to incorporate into your life, for the rest of your life. Take it slowly. Treasure the time you have for yourself. Just winning the mental battle to get out there is the most important thing.

Before I started to run, I did a lot of walking. So you may need to start walking 5km for a week or two first. Get a tracking app for your phone, find a run that you are going to enjoy and map out 5km. I am extremely lucky because I live in Warrandyte and I get to run on the Yarra and in the State Park every day. I started out on a treadmill but found this really boring. Being in nature reduces anger, fear, and stress and increases pleasant feelings. Exposure to nature not only makes you feel better emotionally, it contributes to your physical wellbeing, reducing blood pressure, heart rate, muscle tension, and the production of stress hormones. So exercise outside to get the most from your cardio workout.

When you are ready, build up to the 5km distance by using a run/walk strategy and slowly building up your running intervals and don't go too fast. You may find that you can increase your distance if you just . . . slow . . . down. Move at a conversational pace, which means that you should be able to talk in complete sentences as you're running. If you find yourself getting out of breath, slow it down. As you build your fitness, you'll be able to pick up your pace but, for now, focus on increasing your distance.

Make it fun

I love this time because it is mine. I use it to clear my head and get ready for the day. When I first started running, I felt so good about myself when it was over, but as my fitness has built over time I really enjoy it while I am out there.

I have a playlist, a couple I always play and change the rest according to my mood. I am a bit of a 70s freak and am still in love with Johnny T in *Saturday Night Fever* and *Grease*. Have you ever seen anyone move like him?

Anyway . . . here are some of my faves:
- *Stayin Alive'* – Bee Gees
- *I'm a Believer* – Smash Mouth
- *All Over the World* – ELO
- *September* – Earth, Wind and Fire
- *Amazing* – George Michael
- *Miss Independent* – Kelly Clarkson
- *Lovely Day* – Bill Withers
- *King of Wishful Thinking* – Go West

- *Somebody Like You* – Keith Urban
- *Escaping* – Margaret Urlich
- *Walking on Broken Glass* – Annie Lennox
- *Sing Hallelujah!* – Dr Alban
- *Shivers* – Ed Sheeran

As soon as I hear these songs my brain tells me I need to start running. These are some of my examples but music is such a personal thing, so download music that makes you feel great. Download your favourite songs onto a running playlist, get out there and don't ever give up.

Remember, it's you versus your comfort zone. You can push yourself some days and maybe take it easy on yourself on other days. There are some days I just fly and others where I really struggle. This can depend on a lot of factors (especially what I happened to drink the day before). Some may want to achieve personal bests, others may simply want to jog. Do what is good for you. I have a hill that I use to push myself. It starts at a carpark and takes me up to Pound Bend State Park. I put *Miss Independent* on Spotify and if I make it to the top before the song finishes, I am happy. If I make it to the top with a PB I jump around like Rocky in the scene where he runs up the stairs. It's all about getting out there and having fun.

The other thing I have found is that if something is troubling me, I put it to the back of my mind and by the end of my run I have usually found the answer or know how I am going to deal with it. Running, for just 30 minutes, is such an empowering thing. I hope that you make it part of your life.

Chapter 15

Strength is the new beautiful

Without question, the biggest game changer for me was when I started resistance training. I felt the fittest, strongest and healthiest I have in my whole life when I started to lift weights. It was such an amazing feeling after my first session. I felt like I could do anything. Why didn't I know about this earlier? I so wish that I had. You see, in my teenage world and well into my 30s and 40s, it was all about being as skinny as you possibly could. You know, that lovely emaciated model walking-skeleton look that pushes the mental boundaries of young women over the edge into starving themselves and sometimes causing dangerous eating disorders.

There is a new term being thrown about now, which is 'skinny fat'. It refers to someone who appears thin in size, but their body is mostly fat and has very little muscle. So someone can starve themselves and only do cardio until they become frail and skinny, but because what's left on their fragile skinny body is just skin and fat, it is not healthy. As you become older this becomes more obvious.

I used to think that simply running on the treadmill or the elliptical for 45 minutes was enough, but skipping strength training is a mistake. By ignoring strength training, you are robbing both your bones and muscles of the opportunity to strengthen and grow.

Women's attitudes to their bodies are changing. You can see it all over social media, women are no longer interested in starving themselves to be skinny, they want to build strength and sculpt muscles. They no longer want to be seen as a princess or a damsel in distress, they want to lead empowered lives and this is leading to changes in the way they eat and exercise.

Instagram is arguably the internet's largest platform for fitness models and trainers and these women all have beautifully strong toned bodies. How I wish this cultural shift had happened when I was a teenager.

Strength is beauty. You can't be skinny or underweight and strong. Women are now realising that their body composition – what you are made of – is more important than the number on the scale. Women have avoided lifting heavy weights in the past as they have felt it will make them look masculine, but this is not the case. Women have about 20% less testosterone in their body than men do and without the extra testosterone we are biologically unable to bulk up like men. Personally, I can do the same weights and rep ranges as my husband on legs day (definitely not on arms day) but I will never be able to get as big as him. It makes me strong though and I love feeling strong. I want to make sure when I am older that I am jumping out of my chair, not struggling to get out of it.

Another myth about building muscle and strength is that you have to spend long hard hours in the gym. This is not the case, you simply have to start putting your major muscle groups under pressure with some heavy weights once to twice a week. Your muscles need recovery time so it won't be any more than that.

Seven reasons why muscle increases your beauty and makes you look younger

1. When you build muscle and you strengthen and tone the muscles beneath the skin, you make the skin look healthier. The stronger your muscles are, the more support the skin will have and the firmer and more elastic the skin will look.

2. When you work out, especially when you are building muscle, your blood circulation increases and delivers oxygen and nutrients to your skin cells. Those oxygen and nutrients repair damaged skin, increase collagen production and produce natural oils, so your skin ends up feeling supple and hydrated.

3. Being strong also enhances your life and makes you more functionally fit and capable. Being skinny, if it comes from calorie restriction, under-nutrition and too much aerobic exercise, makes you weaker and less able to do your daily activities without feeling fatigued. Looking tired instead of full of energy is extremely aging.

4. Lifting weights helps to encourage the production of two anti-aging hormones: oxytocin and progesterone. Recent research also shows that working your muscles increases the production of collagen cells and stimulates the production of growth hormone.

5. The Basal Metabolic Rate (BMR) is the rate the body needs in energy (calories) to keep all its systems functioning correctly,

such as breathing, keeping the heart beating to circulate blood, growing and repairing cells and adjusting hormone levels. The body's BMR accounts for the largest amount of energy expended daily (50–80% of your daily energy use). Your BMR is largely determined by your total muscle mass because this requires a lot of energy to maintain. Anything that increases muscle mass will increase your BMR. The more you strength train and the stronger you become, the higher the number of calories you will burn at rest because your metabolism will be fired up. So put simply, the more muscle you have the more calories you will burn at rest, which will naturally reduce the amount of fat you are carrying.

6. Muscle improves our posture, and good posture can make us look younger, thinner and taller. The main cause of poor posture is muscle loss and imbalance. When you engage in strength training you enable your muscles to fine-tune your coordination, appearance, movement and balance. People with great posture generally have a commanding and confident presence.

7. Strength training slows and reverses the aging process at a cellular level. Without trying to sound too scientific, cellular health is linked to mitochondrial health (the powerhouses of cells) and telomere length (chromosomal end caps). Mitochondria increase energy production and also reverse the genetic profile of our DNA. Telomere length actually determines the biological lifespan of an organism.

Building muscle is so important for our longevity. Did you know that according to the Centers for Disease Control and Prevention, falls are the leading cause of injury and death in older Americans? This is a result of reduced muscle strength and decreased activity. After the age of 30, whether you are male or female, you are losing 1% of your muscle mass every single year. Sarcopenia is a condition characterised by loss of skeletal muscle mass and function. If we are talking about longevity, we must look at ways we can build sarcopenia resistance. We want to resist the gradual muscle mass loss over our lifetime. This results in an increased lifespan and also an increase in the quality of our life. Increasing our strength is extraordinarily important to our longevity.

Lifting heavy weights (and getting enough calcium) is also one of the only ways to increase your bone density. So if you don't want brittle bones when you are 70, nothing makes bones stronger than lifting weights.

Fuelling your body properly with nutritious and delicious foods, getting the right amount of rest combined with strength training has extraordinary health and anti-aging benefits. Over time, living a fit and active lifestyle can reverse many of the effects of aging. It will drastically reduce the risk of developing many life-threatening conditions such as osteoporosis, heart disease, type 2 diabetes and Alzheimer's. On top of that you will feel fantastic as you build your self-image, increase your stamina and the mood-boosting endorphins kick in.

In summary, to get the best out of your body and to avoid unnecessary aging and all the pain that comes with it you need to do some strength training, consistently. Weight training is a serious therapy to stop or even reverse the effects of aging. I understand that going to the gym can be pretty scary for the first time, especially if you are the only female in a room full of testosterone. All that equipment looks so complicated but it's not.

Women can have gym anxiety and find them quite intimidating. However, they are very different now and include female personal trainers to take you through how the gym equipment works. They are a lot more female-friendly as women become more aware of how important resistance training is to their physical wellbeing and the results that can be achieved in as little as half an hour twice a week.

Lifting weights will be one of the best things that has ever happened to your fitness routine and your body. When you start to go to the gym and you see your body change it becomes exciting. Even the smallest of changes is empowering because your body is becoming stronger as well as more toned, you can see it and you can feel it. It is simple and it is life-changing.

Chapter 16

My simple resistance training routine

Becoming strong and toned isn't nearly as complicated and difficult as the fitness industry wants you to believe. In fact, it's simple. I have reduced my body fat percentage by 10% and increased my muscle mass by 8% with the routine below that honestly takes me 30 minutes twice a week.

In the previous chapter we established how important resistance training is in the fight against aging because adults lose muscle every decade of their life, which underlines all the perils of aging – osteoporosis, type-2 diabetes, cardiovascular disease, unwanted weight gain, an increased susceptibility to illness and fall-related injuries.

Strength training is the best type of exercise as it is the only one that improves all the key biomarkers of fitness at the same time, such as:

- body composition
- strength and muscle mass
- bone density

- blood pressure
- telomere length
- cardio fitness
- aerobic capacity
- blood glucose control.

Yep, pumping iron offers the best way to increase our longevity and make us look fantastic. But where do you start? How heavy do you need to lift for best gains in muscle and strength? How often? Which machines should you use? How many reps should you do?

The six major muscle groups you want to train are the chest, back, arms, shoulders, legs and calves. I go to the gym for strength training as this is the best place to be and I like to use the machines rather than free weights. One of the main upsides is that the machines are much easier to learn, and you are able to lift heavier weights due to a fixed range of motion which limits usage of other muscle groups. It's much easier to target the muscle groups that you want to work when you are using machines. There is also less chance of injury.

The machines I use at the gym are:
- lat pulldown machine
- chest press
- the seated cable row
- shoulder press
- assisted pull-up machine for biceps
- leg press machine
- Smith machine for squats
- abdominals (optional).

There are other machines you can use to emphasise specific muscles but to keep things quick and simple and still get results, these are the only machines I use.

When you first start resistance training it is very important to make sure you are doing it properly and that you have the right form. Once you have achieved the correct form, then you can play with weight, number of repetitions and rest time.

It is then important to understand the concept of progressive overload, which is when you gradually increase the weight or number of repetitions in your strength training routine. This challenges your body and allows your musculoskeletal system to get stronger.

Doing the same workouts over and over or using the same amount of weights every time you strength train can lead to your body plateauing. You may be able to easily lift weight that once was challenging, and you likely don't notice any soreness or any progress being made. While a plateau can be seen as a positive sign that means you've made some gains in your fitness journey, it also signals that it's time to mix things up.

You can achieve progressive overload in two basic ways, by increasing the number of repetitions or sets you do or by increasing the weight. When you are a beginner it is probably best to first increase the reps, then the number of sets, and then the weight. For example, in the first month of strength training, you might perform 10 repetitions at one weight. Then, the next month, you'd perform 12 reps of the exercise. Later you may go to 10 reps but increase the weight you're using instead.

I have outlined the benefits of each machine below. I have specifically not put in instructions on how to use the equipment as it would be more beneficial for you to be taken through this at the gym with the staff there. As I explained earlier, there are many female personal trainers now available to you at your local gym. Just let them know that these are the pieces of equipment you would like to be shown how to use.

For each exercise I recommend starting with three sets of 10 reps. Start with less if you have to, always listening to your body to avoid injury. The last repetition should always feel difficult.

Rest for a few minutes between sets.

Lat pull-down

Benefits:

The lat pull-down machine is mainly used to exercise your upper back muscles, the lower part and the rhomboids. The lat pull-down is a fantastic exercise to strengthen the latissimus dorsi muscle, the broadest muscle in your back, which promotes good posture and spinal stability.

Training with this machine helps significantly reduce tension on your shoulder and neck area. By isolating the back muscles with this machine, you can focus specifically on your back muscles without tiring out your biceps or triceps.

Chest press
Benefits:

The seated chest press machine is a great exercise as it targets the main muscle of the chest, the pectorals. It also helps build the biceps, triceps and the big muscles of the shoulders and back – the deltoids and the latissimus dorsi (lats). The arms, placed under a weight-bearing load, are pushed away from the chest and returned to starting position.

The seated cable row
Benefits:

The seated cable row is a pulling exercise that works the back muscles in general, particularly the latissimus dorsi. It also works the forearm muscles and the upper arm muscles, as the biceps and triceps are the stabilisers for this exercise.

Shoulder press
Benefits:

This exercise targets several of the major upper body muscles including the deltoids, trapezius, triceps and the upper portion of the pecs. When using a shoulder press machine, you're targeting the large muscle groups like the deltoids with more focus. This means you will be able to lift heavier, as weaker muscles won't stop you performing it.

Assisted pull-up machine for biceps

The pull-up is one of the best exercises for biceps and this is a fantastic machine if you are not up to doing them on your own yet, as it can help you work up to it. In the assisted pull-up, you will select a weight in the weight stack. However, unlike many machines, the higher the weight you select, the easier the exercise will be. This is because the weight that you choose is deducted from your body weight when you do the pull-up.

Leg press

Benefits:

This is a great machine, my favourite. This is the machine to give you stronger, more defined, sexier looking legs. Leg presses are also a great way to strengthen your glutes, which is something that everybody, especially the ladies, want to have because it makes your butt look really nice. The leg press is a compound exercise, which means that it helps to exercise virtually every major muscle and muscle group in your legs at once.

A big benefit of using a leg press machine is that depending on what position your feet and legs are in, different leg muscles will be worked to a different degree; this allows you to focus on a specific muscle group to achieve the best results possible.

For example, if you place your feet near the top of the platform you will be focusing more on your hamstrings and glutes. On the other hand, if you put your feet lower on the platform, you will be focusing more on your quadriceps. You can also move your feet so that your heels are not on the platform at all, and so you are only using the balls of your feet and toes to lift the weight, and this will focus on your calves.

Smith machine squats

Benefits:

Your lower body boasts some of your largest and most powerful muscles. From getting out of bed, to sitting down in a chair, your glutes, quadriceps, hamstrings, adductors, hip flexors and calves are responsible for almost every move you make. Squats will help strengthen and tone all of these muscles in your lower body.

The Smith machine allows you to protect your shoulders, legs, knees and back from injury. You are also able to more efficiently engage your glutes and hamstrings. Using this machine helps you to avoid some of the injuries associated with free squats.

Abs

Yes, tight, toned abs look amazing. But their health benefits are even better.

A strong core protects your back and spine, preventing injury. Because many of your body's movements originate from your core, working toward improving its strength will enhance your posture, spinal alignment, stability, protect against back pain, protect your inner organs and more.

Weightlifting will definitely strengthen your core so you may choose not to add extra abdominal exercises. However, ab specific exercises can help make your abs even stronger and help with that six-pack if that is what you are after.

I do 15–20 reps of each exercise (one after the other), referred to as a superset. Do the superset three times. It should take about

15 minutes. When I am working on my abdominals, I try to do this two to three times a week. My superset includes:

- ab crunch with weight
- seated rotation
- cross toe touch
- bicycle twist
- mountain climbers.

Demonstrations of these ab exercises can easily be found if you search them on YouTube.

In general, weight machines are a great tool for beginners, as they teach proper form and reduce the risk of injury. You can complete a full-body circuit by choosing half a dozen body machines, and many machines will have instructions on the frame, giving you a step-by-step idea of how it works and the muscles you'll be target-ing. Remember, if you're unsure, there is always someone who works at the gym you can ask for help, and more often than not these days, females are the PT who will be helping you.

I love machines as they are easy to use, specific, safe and it is simple and quick to increase the weights as I feel I need to. They are all I need to feel strong and toned.

Before I finish this chapter however, it would be remiss of me not to mention free weights. This means you will be using dumb-bells, barbells, or kettlebells to perform the exercise. Free weights engage more muscles as your body stabilises itself; it is however extremely important to make sure your form is correct. As your muscles start to tire it is easy to lose form. If you are going to use free weights I would suggest that you definitely engage a trainer. As you become stronger you may want to incorporate both into your routine.

In short, strength training means slowing and reversing the aging process at the cellular and genetic level. It increases your energy, improves brain function and protects against disease. Without question it is the most powerful solution we have at our disposal in our battle against time. The results we need to age successfully are all about the pursuit and production of increased strength.

It is very easy to incorporate into your life just by using some simple machines at the gym. Get a friend or an accountability partner to start with you, but just do whatever it takes to make resistance training an important part of your weekly routine.

Section 5
The pursuit of the ageless face

The aim of this section is to show the changing (or should I say unchanging) face of the future. We don't have to age the way we once did and it doesn't need to be secret women's business either. There is now a much greater open-mindedness around the topics of botox, laser treatments and surgery. The normalisation of these procedures will mean that we can discuss openly each type of procedure, what it can achieve, the price and if it is the right thing for you depending on what you would like to achieve.

The right knowledge is so empowering and there are so many options available to us now. It is exciting as our options are constantly increasing as technology advances and prices continually decrease.

Chapter 17

My journey to creating skincare that works

Where it all began

My story starts in the Australian Outback city of Broken Hill, in Northwest New South Wales – the birthplace of 'The Big Australian', BHP (Broken Hill Proprietary), and I am proud to say, myself.

BHP was a turning point in the creation of wealth for this incredible country. Although many of us only know Broken Hill as the place where *Mad Max* and *The Adventures of Priscilla, Queen of the Desert* were filmed, it is so much more. I don't understand why a film has not been made about the rags-to-riches story of the 14 original founders of BHP. The story of the quiet, balding, boundary rider Charles Rasp, who in 1883 discovered a treasure trove that was a rich, deep and wide ore body. And the story of the unimaginable wealth that this discovery brought to them all. Maybe one day the film will be made ...

Not only has Broken Hill made huge contributions to the wealth, welfare and social structure of Australia, but at the turn of the twentieth century, it also led the world in mining and minerals processing technology. A London newspaper described 'The Big Mine' as the best-managed in the world, and by 1907 there were 5000 on the payroll.

One of those employees was my Great Grandfather, Alfred Hocking. He was the fourth person (of 800) to die working underground, at the age of 28. The conditions were extremely dangerous, and as a result, in 1917, after many years of uprisings by the unions, the 35-hour work week and better working conditions were born.

Living in Broken Hill was still very difficult at that time, despite what the unions had achieved. Working conditions were extremely haphazard, and living conditions above ground were very poor.

My Grandpa spent his working life underground and, after hours, at one of the many pubs (as most of the miners did), while my Grandma raised a family of five in a miner's shack.

My resentful Grandma was very unhappy and scary to me at the age of six. She barely tolerated me as a young child. I thought she was like this because of the deeply engraved lines on her face and the stooped way she walked. I didn't understand at the time; the real reason was a life of hardship that had worn her down.

For my generation, though, Broken Hill had become an amazing place to grow up. The living conditions had vastly improved. My Dad was an accountant for the mining company CRA, and after hours he was the singer in a band. Mum was a secretary at the hospital and was also a model in the local paper. We had so much fun with our family and friends, even if there was only one park that had grass where we could go for a picnic.

What a place to spend your childhood – no crime, no locked doors. Everyone looked out for each other and everybody laughed. It was a place where you could safely pretend to be your own superhero when playing in the dusty backyard (although one day Mum had to put a stop to me jumping off the Hills Hoist clothesline). My superpower was going to be not getting old and unhappy like Grandma. So, with the innocence and adventurous spirit of a child, I decided I would do whatever it took to prevent being miserable like that when I grew older.

I was an absolute tomboy with short hair – the only time I ever wore a dress was to church on Sundays. But I so desperately wanted to do anything that would make me look pretty. I would make Mum put curlers in my short hair, even though they would fall out and do absolutely nothing to help me look like my best friend, who had beautiful long curly hair.

And then it happened – one day, I was sitting on the floor watching our black-and-white TV, and an advertisement came on. A beautiful woman getting off a train, the camera panned to the handsome husband waiting for her. She ran to him, and they embraced, and then the next thing you saw was a glass jar filled with a miracle face cream.

In my mind, it was the answer to not growing old (and unhappy like Grandma), and it was the beginning of my quest. That's where and why my skincare obsession started.

Finding the answer

While the deep lines etched into my Grandma's face, representing a life of utter hardship, is an extreme example, I learned at an early age that there is a deep connection between how we look and how we feel.

That TV advertisement changed everything in my young mind. I went straight to my Mum's bathroom to see if she already had this miracle cure but couldn't find anything – just the normal things like soap and a hairbrush.

And then I started to nag her. Please, could she buy some? Mum was curious as to why I kept insisting, but said she would try to find it for me. None could be found anywhere in Broken Hill, which didn't surprise me.

Mum promised she would look for it next time she was in Adelaide, the closest major city, seven hours' drive away. I couldn't wait. A couple of months later, Mum returned from Adelaide with the cream but said that it was ridiculous to be using it at my age. She started using it herself, which meant I could use it when she wasn't looking.

This obsession did not leave me. Dad's company relocated us to Melbourne, and I was able to get my first part-time job as a 'checkout chick' at Target. This meant I could now purchase my own creams. I would spend hours in the chemist investigating the latest brands and deciding which one I should buy. I ended up trying them all. While I spent some time in my teenage years on the problem of how to blow-dry my hair to stop it from being frizzy (still a problem) and how to apply eyeliner correctly, my obsession with skincare continued.

When I finished Year 12, I took a 'gap year' and worked at the ANZ Bank, which meant I could afford the latest and greatest brands like Clinique. I will never forget the time I first pulled that beautiful square glass jar out of its light-green box, the silver lid, and the light-yellow colour of the cream.

I finished up at the bank and started to study for my bachelor's degree in Accounting. I supported myself by selling … guess what … skincare! After only six months, I was one of the top-performing sales reps for Nutrimetics, which was a new brand that had just exploded onto the Australian scene.

After I had finished my tertiary studies, and with the newfound income from embarking on my accounting career, I could afford to try the skincare ranges available at David Jones department store. This was the time I started to ask some questions, probably because my skin was now starting to show some signs of aging. Which one should I buy, how much should I spend, and what is it actually doing for my skin?

I have watched the skincare industry evolve and explode with great fascination. And I would have to say, confusion. I would guess that many are the same. When I walk into stores like Sephora and Mecca and I ask the salesgirls what I should be using, I think I end up being even more confused than when I walked in.

Some brands promote a 10-step process (this is the Korean way) — even as an avid skincare enthusiast, it's not something I think is necessary and, to be honest, I just don't have the time.

My curiosity had not subsided at all since the age of six. So, I started to read everything I could find on skincare. What ingredients worked and why? What percentage of active ingredients should we use? Are natural ingredients as potent as those from the lab?

How could I truly investigate this?

At this stage, I had built a very successful finance business, and my three boys were now young men. It was my time. Time to pursue my dreams and passions. So, I decided to sell my business so I could concentrate on writing my book and creating the skincare I wanted.

Of course, this was going to be much easier said than done. Where would I even start?

Have you heard the saying 'ask the universe and you will find the answer'?

When a very dear friend of mine realised that this was the path I was now taking, she connected me with an expat she had studied with in Europe who had just developed a skincare range in Paris. This was the beginning of an amazing journey for me. I spent the next year talking to manufacturers, ingredient suppliers and formulators. What I eventually found out over that year was I had opened Pandora's box. There was so much more I needed to learn, and the place to do that was at the biggest beauty trade show in the world, Cosmoprof, held every year in Bologna.

Why not? I would fly to Bologna and find the definitive answers there.

Bologna has been hosting the world's largest beauty trade show for over 50 years. It is the food capital of Italy and boasts the longest porticos anywhere in the world. It has a population of 380,000 but when the trade show starts, it has an extra 250,000 visitors over a four-day period. It is next to impossible to get accommodation or a cab. Most people train it in from Florence or Milan. The exhibition grounds are beyond huge. It is 160,000 square metres (or 40 acres) and has 3000 exhibitors from 64 countries.

It was overwhelming, but for me, it was just a bigger version of all the research I had been doing in stores since I was six.

I walked approximately 30,000 steps every day for four days, visiting as many stands as possible and asking as many questions as I could.

I was scared that the exhibitors would not be bothered with me, but this was not the case at all. In fact, it was exactly the opposite. They loved that I had travelled from Australia (there was only one Australian stand there), and they were beyond helpful, giving me as much information as they possibly could. The show covered everything: the latest trends and innovations, raw ingredients, manufacturing solutions, formulators, scientific breakthroughs, and packaging.

I remember the very last day of that trade show, walking out of the building. It was a freezing cold day, but there was not a drop of wind or a cloud in the sky. I had the sun on my face and excitement in my heart because I had found my answer.

While I was standing in that beautiful Italian city, I realised the answer, unbelievably, was back home, where it all began.

Fifty years on, I had travelled and researched endlessly, spoken to the best cosmetic chemists and scientists around the world, and the answer was in Broken Hill. How could I ever have known it was at the feet of that six-year-old girl?

The making of the cream

For me, the formula I needed to create was one that would deliver clinically proven, noticeable and highly effective results, provide an extremely sensory experience, contain the highest quality ingredients, and be simple – not an overly complicated and unnecessary regimen. Warning: there is a lot of information here – but I think it is very important for me to include the *hows* and *whys* I used to create something beautiful that you can trust.

There are five major areas we have addressed when creating our formulation, as explained below.

1. Nature vs science

Today, the gap between natural products and scientific advancements is closing. Formulators and Cosmetic Scientists create products that are no longer restricted to one approach. Instead, they use the newest findings and technologies from both nature and our laboratories. These are no longer mutually exclusive. Nature is science, and we will be sourcing our ingredients from an innovative supplier that leads the way in the cellular extraction of compounds from our great Australian biodiversity and practices conscious and sustainable manufacturing.

This brings me to our native hero ingredient which grows prolifically in Broken Hill, where I would run through it barefoot as a little girl – who would have ever thought: the Australian desert saltbush.

Australian desert saltbush contains potent compounds beneficial for skin health, particularly in slowing the aging process. Here's why it is considered so powerful:

- *Adaptation to harsh habitats:* The desert saltbush has developed potent antioxidants as a defence against its arid, saline environment. These antioxidants combat free radicals, which cause skin aging.
- *High mineral content:* The plant contains minerals such as zinc and selenium, which are essential for skin health, contributing to improved elasticity and fewer wrinkles. It is also rich in calcium, magnesium, iron and potassium, which support skin hydration and barrier function.
- *Unique phytochemicals:* The desert saltbush produces various phytochemicals in response to its environment, which have numerous benefits for the skin, including improved permeability, vitality, elasticity, lightening effects, reduced pigment production and anti-aging properties. They also have anti-inflammatory and antimicrobial activities and stimulate collagen and elastin synthesis.
- *Hydration retention:* Adapted to retain moisture, the desert saltbush may transfer these hydrating properties to the skin, aiding in moisture retention and barrier maintenance, especially beneficial for dry skin.

Additionally, desert saltbush contains beta-carotene, a vitamin A precursor, which helps maintain skin health, improve appearance, repair tissues, and protect against sun damage.

Australian Desert Saltbush also contains high amounts of Protocatechuic Acid (PCA), which has outstanding skin permeability. This brings me to the next important factor in our formulation.

2. Permeation of the skin

The efficacy of a formulation is determined not only by its ingredients but also by its ability to permeate the skin's barrier.

Permeation is the process by which the active ingredients in topical cosmetic products pass through the skin. We want to ensure that when we apply a formulation to our skin, the ingredients don't just sit on the surface; they actually move through the skin's outer layer, the stratum corneum, to reach the inner layers where they can have a beneficial effect.

Cosmetic chemists aim to improve how well the active ingredients are delivered to the target site within the skin. For example, to stimulate collagen production – a key biological process for maintaining skin's elasticity and youthfulness – it's essential that the ingredients can get past the tough outer layer of the skin. The selection of our active ingredients is based on their molecular size and their specific ability to permeate this barrier to ensure their effectiveness.

3. The skin barrier (the epidermis or outer layer)

While permeation of the skin's outer layer is a key component, the ingredients need to protect, calm and improve the skin's barrier.

The skin barrier is like a shield that keeps out harmful substances like pollution and germs, while also retaining hydration. It also helps to keep your skin moist and healthy. If it gets damaged by pollution, rough skin treatments, strong soaps, poor nutrition, dehydration, hormonal changes or aging, your skin can become dry and irritated, heal slowly, and become more prone to developing blemishes or other skin problems.

It is crucial not to break down or inflame the skin's outer layer when using skincare products. When our skin becomes irritated, it triggers the release of agents that can cause inflammatory damage and destruction of the skin's structural components, including collagen and elastin, which can contribute to wrinkle formation.

Overuse of active ingredients and excessive use of strong skincare products can also compromise this shield, especially products meant to exfoliate or renew the skin, such as retinoids and acids. While these can help make your skin appear smoother and younger, excessive use can strip away the skin's natural oils and moisture, leading to irritation and dryness. Therefore, it's important to be cautious with these products, observe how your skin reacts to them, and use products that help repair and moisturise the skin to maintain its strength and health.

4. We do not need to apply actives separately

I could not tell you the number of times I have walked into a skincare store or department or visited a website and thought, 'This is crazy. What do I do here? What should I buy?'

When creating AIJAN, I wanted to make sure it was a simple and comprehensive solution. I wanted to make sure it would be considered the brand for successful, discerning women who want simple, premium skincare that has been proven to work, so they can be confident in making the right choice.

Many of our competitors push a diverse number of products to capitalise on the latest trends, which can be extraordinarily confusing and overwhelming. We are taking the confusion out of skincare by offering a fully comprehensive, luxury and clinically proven formulation.

The ingredients in our BMPC formulation (patent-pending) will address all skincare needs, including:

- *Skin elasticity*: plumpness and bounce back of the skin
- *Skin laxity*: volume and firmness
- *Skin smoothness*: drastic reduction of wrinkles
- *Skin inflammation*: calm and reduce redness
- *Skin hyperpigmentation*: dark spots/age spots visibly reduce
- *Skin hydration*: deep tissue hydration

We have created a beautiful, rich, thick cream that melts immediately into the skin and has clinically proven highly effective results in one product.

5. Trust is key – why clinical testing matters

I believe that transparency and ethical practices are fundamental in building trust within this industry.

Clinical trials are crucial in the beauty sector, ensuring that skincare is effective and safe for use. These tests carefully evaluate new product formulas and components on volunteers, gathering important information about their impact and any associated risks.

Results need to be proven on the combination of ingredients, the formulation, not just on one ingredient alone.

Our trials scientifically test for moisturizing capabilities, wrinkle reduction and skin texture enhancement. They also test for any possible side effects or allergic responses, confirming the product's safety for buyers.

When we conduct clinical trials, we not only want to ensure that our products meet the highest standards but also push the boundaries of beauty science, setting higher benchmarks for the industry and improving consumer offerings.

* * *

Clearly, the path to create a product like AIJAN was not an easy one. In many ways, it's been a lifetime in the making for me; I just didn't realise it at the time.

So, what's next?

The journey continues

Today, I draw on my early life. I have great respect for the wild and the gifts it gives us, as well as the people who have lived on this land for tens of thousands of years before us. I believe that the greatest path forward is the one where we reflect deeply on the wisdom of those who came before us. Australia is extraordinary, where the ancient and the modern tell two stories. How wonderful would it be to bring them together and tell a new story, a new way forward?

No matter where my world may be heading, my soul remembers the feel of the red soil, the colour of the sky, and the simplicity of life in the wild place where it all began.

I cannot see my lifelong passion fading, my passion for living a long, happy and fulfilled life. I believe that as we move forward, taking care of ourselves both internally and externally will no longer be seen as something superficial, but as an essential component in increasing our emotional and mental health as we strive for longevity and quality of life. I learned this very early in life, through the eyes of a six-year-old girl staring at her grandmother's face.

Chapter 18

The incredible injectables

There is no question, botox and fillers have absolutely taken the world by storm. Botox and fillers are both great treatments for anti-aging, reducing the appearance of wrinkles and plumping the skin. However, they do different things – while botox keeps wrinkles and fine lines from forming by relaxing the muscles surrounding targeted areas, fillers fill wrinkles and plump desired areas of the face, such as the cheeks and lips.

Outside of having plastic surgery, botox is pretty much the most effective way to reduce the appearance of crow's feet, frown lines and forehead lines. Another key use of botox, which has become increasingly popular in recent years, is the ability to reshape your face. Forget what you used to think about botox. Once considered to be used only by celebrities and the wealthy with a bad rap for freezing faces, these injections have become a commonplace activity.

Botox and fillers used to be only for Boomers, but not any more, as increasingly younger people are embracing the injections. Millennials and Gen Xers are heading to plastic surgeons or dermatologists to prevent their skin from aging. *Forbes* magazine recently reported the use of botox among people aged 19–34 has risen by 87% over the past five years.

Prevention is not the only reason driving the younger people of our population to use injectables. They have a different attitude towards these procedures. The younger generation ask why we are so prejudiced against anti-aging procedures such as botox and fillers when society seems to think it is perfectly okay to spend hundreds of dollars having your hair dyed, cut and blow-dried?

Another driving force behind these procedures in the young is the pressure to look great on social media. A quick search of #botox turns up almost 10.3 million Instagram posts and there are 2.8 million posts for #fillers. With the takeover of the selfie, younger women are getting fillers because they want Kylie Jenner lips, the perfect pout or they want their face to look more like photos created by Snapchat filters. There has been a huge increase in non-surgical procedures for the 19–34 year-olds which coincides with the growing selfie obsession and use of social media filters.

So is this for you? Knowing the differences between botox and filler and their purposes as well as being aware of what you would like to achieve is essential in picking the right treatment for you.

Botox

I love botox. Love it, love it, love it. It has been an absolute game changer for my face. It is an amazing rejuvenator. It fits into my busy life because the treatments are quick and convenient. Most people are good candidates for the treatment because it's suitable for the majority of healthy adults. Both men and women regularly get botox, since wrinkles affect everyone. It is minimally invasive and affordable compared to many other procedures.

I first started using botox when I was about 40. I have it where my frown lines are and also for crow's feet. Not only has this stopped wrinkles, it has had other benefits for me as it has stopped the consistent headaches I always had in this area. If I had known that, I would have started using it much earlier. Having botox for my frown lines has also opened up my eyes, like a semi-brow lift. As I said earlier, I love it.

Botox is made from a purified protein that relaxes wrinkles and rejuvenates the appearance of the face. It can literally make you look years younger after one treatment. You can immediately experience smoother skin, elevated brows and a more youthful appearance in a matter of minutes. There is no downtime and you can return to your normal activities immediately following the procedure.

Botox works by reducing the muscle's ability to contract fully, thereby reducing or removing the wrinkle. The lack of muscle contraction prevents the face from forming or deepening lines and wrinkles so it is also preventative. The result is smoother skin until it wears off. The effects of botox are visible two to 10 days after treatment and last about three to six months, depending on the person and how many treatments they have had. It is more common for effects to last longer after multiple treatments.

Botox removes wrinkles in the following areas by using a very fine needle to inject it into the selected facial muscles. Discomfort is minimal and brief, there is a quick sting which lasts for a few seconds and this can even be further reduced by making the area cold first.

Botox is used for:

- frown lines between the eyebrows
- lines across the bridge of the nose
- forehead lines
- 'crow's feet' wrinkles extending from the outside corners of the eyes
- lines on the throat (turkey neck).

While botox is generally thought of as a procedure that smooths fine lines and softens wrinkles, it is also useful for changing the face. Here are some of the things it can do to change the shape of your face without surgery.

Slim the face

If you would like a slimmer, more oval-shaped face, botox can do this for you by having it injected into the masseter muscles. These are the muscles located at the back of the jaw, which can be overactive, so this can also help with teeth grinding and jaw clenching as well. Botox can relax these muscles, which will reduce their activity and reduce their size. With botox in the masseter muscles, you can see a dramatic change in the contours of your face and if you are a teeth grinder it will stop that as well.

Alter your jawline

Just as botox can slim your face, often with an injection into the masseter muscles, it is possible to exaggerate the jawline by adding more firmness to an undefined jaw. This is a common procedure for men as a strong, square-shaped jawline is a traditionally attractive feature in males. A few strategically placed injections of botox can not only increase jaw definition but can also firm up or change the shape of the chin. This is also a great way to tighten jowls. If your jawline has become less defined, a little botox along the muscles of the jawbone can pull the skin up for a more defined effect.

Lift your lips

You can also achieve those Kylie Jenner youthful-looking lips with botox by injecting tiny drops of it along the upper lip border in order to roll the top lip up and out slightly so it appears plumper. It's subtler than fillers, and because the technique requires less botox than other areas of the face, it's also less expensive.

Change the shape of your nose

I know it is depressing but at about 40 your nose can begin to sag which can make your whole face appear droopy. Botox can help by lifting the nose and taking off years in about 10 minutes. Injecting botox at the base of the nose (between the nostrils) releases the depressor muscle that pulls the nose downward, making the whole face appear more lifted.

Many people want to change the shape or size of their nose, rhinoplasty (commonly known as a nose job) is one of the most popular plastic surgeries of the face. I have had three surgeries on my nose which I will talk further about in Chapter 20 – believe me, they are not fun. It is a major surgery, which requires anesthesia and a long downtime period. You really don't want to see anyone after rhinoplasty!

Botox (and fillers) can be a great alternative depending on what you would like to do. An experienced professional can change the shape of your nose, fix bumps, straighten a crooked appearance, change the shape of the tip, and stop flaring nostrils with simple, non-invasive injections and minimal downtime.

And the miracle of botox continues. It is currently one of the most studied chemical compounds by the medical profession and is being used for many medical reasons such as migraines, depression, chronic pain, bladder disorders and eye spasms.

This is an extract from an article in *Time* magazine:

> Now, thanks in large part to off-label use, Botox – the wrinkle smoother that exploded as a cultural phenomenon and medical triumph – is increasingly being drafted for problems that go far beyond the cosmetic. The depression suffered by Rosenthal's patient is just one example on a list that includes everything from excessive sweating and neck spasms to leaky bladders, premature ejaculation, migraines, cold hands and even the dangerous cardiac condition of atrial fibrillation after heart surgery, among others. The range of conditions for which doctors are now using Botox is dizzying, reflecting the drug's unique characteristics as much as the drug industry's unique strategies for creating a blockbuster.

For all these reasons botox is one of the most popular cosmetic treatments available on the market. It is relatively inexpensive and has little or no recovery time. In fact, you can get it done at lunchtime and then head straight back to work with incredible results.

So why, when botox is more popular than ever before, is it continuously portrayed in a negative light?

Let's dispel some of the myths.

Some think that botox will give them a frozen expression. A botox injection is extremely localised, meaning it affects only the muscles near your wrinkles/fine lines. Botox does not impact muscles elsewhere on the face, and it doesn't impact your ability to make a wide variety of smiles and facial expressions. The goal of botox treatment is to smooth out wrinkles and help the person look refreshed, not emotionless. Unless you have too much botox too frequently, this will not happen.

There is also a myth that botox is addictive. There is no scientific basis for the idea that botox is addictive. It contains no addictive substances and has no physical properties that would make a person become dependent on it. You may want to continue to have it because you love the way it has made you look and feel, but how is this any different from wearing nice clothes or going to the hairdresser when you need a regrowth touch-up?

Another myth is that botox injections are painful. Most individuals have some minor discomfort. Botox injections are given with extremely fine needles, which means there may be a pinch when the needle is first inserted into the skin, but beyond that the discomfort is minimal.

Botox continues to have a bad reputation because it is sometimes referred to as a poisonous toxin. But while it is a neurotoxin, it is certainly not poisonous. Botox has been FDA-approved since 1989 and cleared for cosmetic use since 2002. Millions of individuals have safely received botox treatment. It is very important, however, that both botox and fillers are administered by a qualified medical professional or injector as they have a full understanding of the anatomy of the face.

My last comment on botox is that it will not get rid of all the wrinkles on your face. Botox is effective in the treatment of dynamic wrinkles, explained in Chapter 17. They are caused by movement.

Fillers

Fillers are different to botox in that they are used for plumping and filling deep lines. Dermal fillers are gel-like substances that are injected beneath the skin to increase facial volume, smooth lines and creases, and/or enhance facial contours. They work very well when they are injected by a professional with a practised eye and detailed knowledge of facial anatomy.

There are different types of dermal fillers available and they are categorised by the substance they contain. Fillers vary in their texture, density, and injection depth. Certain fillers may work better for certain areas than others. Your medical expert will determine which filler is best for you. Generally, softer fillers are used in the lips and sturdier products for cheekbone enhancement. It is important to discuss this with a qualified professional before you proceed.

Fillers are temporary or permanent in nature. As a personal choice I would never have a permanent filler – what if you don't like the result? When filler is used in the right place it can give you instant results smoothing the skin and replacing lost volume, but what if it is overdone? It may make you look puffy and distorted. Hyaluronic acid fillers can be completely dissolved and reversed if you don't like the results.

Permanent fillers were the only ones available decades ago so they were the only option. If something went wrong, if they were injected poorly or became infected, the only way to remove them was with surgery so they are far more limited in use now.

The most common fillers are as follows.

Hyaluronic acid

I have discussed this earlier as it is also used in many creams and serums. Hyaluronic acid is a naturally-occurring substance found in the body. It helps your cells retain moisture, making your skin appear hydrated, plump, and healthy. Hyaluronic acid fillers are usually soft and gel-like. Results are temporary, lasting from six to 12 months.

Calcium hydroxylapatite

A well-known brand for this type of filler is Radiesse.

Calcium hydroxylapatite is one of the most well-studied dermal fillers worldwide and has been substantially used for the correction of more severe facial lines and folds as well as lost volume due to aging. It is found naturally in human bones and is a mineral-like compound. These are temporary fillers which are soft and gel-like but have a thicker consistency than hyaluronic acid fillers, meaning they will last longer. Typically, they last 12 months.

Calcium hydroxylapatite also helps stimulate natural collagen production, and is typically used for deeper lines and wrinkles.

Polylactic acid

A popular brand for these types of fillers is Sculptra.

This type of dermal filler is known as a stimulator as when it is injected into your face as it causes your body's own production of collagen. It is not a wrinkle filler but a volumiser or activator that stimulates the body to produce collagen at the injection sites. This substance is unlike other dermal fillers because it doesn't produce immediate results. Instead, it stimulates your own body's collagen production, so results appear gradually over a period of a few months. This type of dermal filler is considered semi-permanent and can last up to two years but may require two or three visits.

As permanent fillers are being used less and less by the cosmetic industry and not recommended by plastic surgeons in most cases, I won't list them here.

When you have dermal fillers the improvement in your facial contours are evident immediately. They improve your appearance in a very subtle way if done correctly. If done well, you will look like a new, improved version of yourself. Here are some of the ways that they can improve your appearance.

Volumise lips

Plumping the lips is probably the most well-known use for fillers. This is most likely due to celebrities who we think may take it a little too far, like Goldie Hawn's character Elise in the *First Wives*

Club, which was hilarious. Despite being associated with over-filling, lip treatments can achieve a subtle enhancement to the natural shape of the lips and provide a beautiful result. I haven't had my lips volumised or plumped but I have had filler injected along my upper lip line, which I like as it provides definition.

Plump cheeks

Dermal fillers can be used to shape, volumise and enhance cheeks. Lost volume occurs with aging and may contribute to flattening of facial contours. Fillers can be used to restore this lost volume. Enhancing cheek volume can also help with facial balance and proportions. You can also support the lower eyelid by volumising the upper cheek. Filler placed just under the lower eyelid in the upper cheek helps to support the lower eyelid and reduces the appearance of eyebags or hollows under the eye.

Fill in forehead lines

Botox can treat the dynamic wrinkles in our forehead, however, fillers may be required to reduce the appearance of the static lines visible even when the face is at rest. The injections do this by filling in the lines with the hyaluronic acid, which is an already naturally occurring part of the skin.

Reshape the chin or nose

Earlier in this chapter I explained how botox can help reshape the nose. Fillers are also commonly used as a nonsurgical option to reshape areas such as the chin, jawline or nose. It is being referred to as the nonsurgical nose job. This can improve your side profile and reduce the appearance of a sagging neck. In some cases, fillers have eliminated the need for surgical procedures to fix these common complaints.

Eliminate marionette lines

Marionette lines are facial wrinkles that occur with natural aging. The lines run vertically between the mouth and chin, which can also create sagging in the lower half of your face. Dermal filler can provide support for the area to reduce the appearance of the lines. Treatment of the marionette area can lift the mouth corners and prevent the downturning of the mouth which can give a glum appearance to the lower face. This can instantly take years off your age and restore balance with the rest of the face.

Nasolabial folds

Often referred to as smile lines, nasolabial folds are the lines seen from the sides of nose to the corners of the mouth. This area can be corrected with filler to create a softer, youthful and more natural look to the face.

Reduce appearance of scars

Dermal fillers can be used to treat depressed acne scars and other indented forms of scars. Dermal fillers will help to raise the indentations and volume loss caused by acne, creating a smoother appearance.

Chapter 19

Non-surgical treatments

Some wrinkles may be too deep to fix with creams and the time may have come where you need treatments for skin resurfacing. You may feel that your skin needs treatments that are not only topical in nature and this will require devices and treatments that can penetrate the more superficial layers of the skin but are not invasive. The deeper the wrinkles, the more aggressive the treatment may need to be as the treatment will need to penetrate to the deeper levels of the skin.

Or do you find yourself gently pulling back the skin on your face when you look in the mirror and wishing it would stay there? While surgery will give you the most dramatic results, there are other skin tightening and lifting options. If you are looking for facelift results in a jar, this just won't happen. While creams can be preventative and are wonderful for the skin's texture and plumpness, they will not lift sagging skin.

Skin resurfacing treatments

Skin resurfacing treatments help to restore a more youthful, beautiful complexion by removing the most damaged outer layers of skin to reveal the healthier looking skin beneath. They also encourage new, healthy skin cell growth. There are a variety of techniques for skin resurfacing treatments for different types of skin concerns including wrinkles, scars, age spots and discoloration. For maximum effect these sorts of treatments are generally done a few times over a three-month period. I will go through each treatment and what you can expect to achieve.

Microneedling

Microneedling is a minimally invasive cosmetic procedure that's used to treat skin concerns by increasing collagen production. It is also known as collagen induction therapy. The pinpricks from the procedure cause slight injury to the skin and then the skin responds by making new collagen-rich tissue. It helps to eliminate fine lines and wrinkles by using the skin's natural healing abilities and produces collagen and elastin. The pinpricks created during the treatment also allow for greater absorption of creams and serums. A topical numbing cream is applied to ensure the procedure is comfortable.

This can be combined with PRP or what is known as the Vampire facial. In the lead-up to her wedding to Kanye West, Kim Kardashian West shared a video on social media undergoing this procedure. PRP refers to Platelet Rich Plasma which is created by separating platelet plasma from a small sample of your blood, which also helps to produce collagen and elastin.

After the treatment your skin will look quite pink and feel a little rough for a couple of days and you can expect to see results in a couple of weeks as the complexion appears more plump and nourished with the new collagen in the skin cells. It is a good treatment to start after the age of 30 as this is when the skin stops producing new collagen and costs can vary from $400 to $800 per treatment.

Microdermabrasion

Microdermabrasion is a powerful way to exfoliate the skin, while microneedling stimulates the skin. While microdermabrasion treats the skin's surface, the microneedling process reaches deeper layers of the skin. Microdermabrasion can be similar to a light chemical peel. It is a minimally invasive skin treatment that buffs away the outermost layer of the skin. Often several treatments are needed to obtain the required results. A diamond tipped applicator is used to polish the top layer of skin cells. This clears congestion and promotes the growth of healthy new skin cells, often leaving clients feeling smoother, fresher and brighter immediately after treatment.

There is minimal downtime and a treatment will generally cost $150–$200.

Chemical peels

Chemical peels are great for skin resurfacing. They basically remove the top layers of skin from the face and are a deep form of exfoliation. It is a procedure in which a chemical solution is applied to the skin. The stronger the chemical agent being used, the deeper the penetration will be. The skin that grows back is smoother.

There are three types of peels, light, medium and deep. The deeper you go with a chemical peel, the longer the recovery time and the greater the cost will be. Deep peels would need to be done under anesthetic by your doctor, whereas light peels are relatively painless and can be done at a skin clinic with little recovery time. With a light peel, you may need to undergo the procedure more than once to get the desired results.

IPL

This type of treatment is for those brown spots on your face or decolletage that all of sudden start to look darker once you head past 30.

IPL stands for Intense Pulsed Light Therapy. IPL is similar to a laser treatment. However, a laser focuses just one wavelength of light at your skin, while IPL releases light of many different wavelengths.

IPL penetrates down to the second layer of your skin, the dermis, without harming the top layer, the epidermis, so it causes less damage to your skin. Pigment cells in your skin absorb the light energy, which is converted into heat. The heat destroys the unwanted pigment to clear up freckles and other spots. It is used to treat skin discoloration and brown spots and is good for evening out skin tone. IPL requires approximately four to six treatments and there is minimal discomfort and downtime.

IPL ranges in price from $150 to $300 per treatment.

Lasers

Alongside injectables, lasers are among the most popular non-surgical treatments for improving the skin's appearance. There are so many lasers now that can treat a wide range of concerns and as technology continues to evolve more and more are being launched onto the market. Laser resurfacing can decrease the appearance of fine lines, treat loss of skin tone and improve your complexion if you have scars or sun damage. Laser resurfacing can't eliminate excessive or sagging skin though.

Lasers can also remove unwanted hair, acne, scars, skin cancers, tattoos, blood vessels, stretch marks, age spots and psoriasis.

There are basically two types of lasers used for cosmetic skin treatments, ablative and non-ablative. Ablative lasers remove or vaporise the top layer of skin, while non-ablative lasers work by targeting specific cells in the deeper layers of the skin without damaging the top layers. The Fraxel laser is the best type of non-ablative laser currently available. These types of lasers are replacing medium to deep chemical peels because of their effectiveness without causing major damage to the surface levels of the skin and therefore there is less recovery time. The Fraxel laser has become well known as it has been made popular by Kim Kardashian. It is probably the best laser for wrinkle removal, treatment of crow's feet, sun damage removal and overall skin rejuvenation. Fraxel can really give you some amazing results. It's a resurfacing laser that enhances the natural healing response of the skin and cellular turnover, resulting in plump, dewy skin.

There is some downtime with Fraxel, but after three to four days looking like you have been sunburned your skin will look years younger, tighter and be completely refreshed. The results are immediate, however your skin continues to improve over the next three to six months as the deeper layers of the skin continue to create new collagen. The number of treatments you require will vary according to the current condition of your skin and what you would like to achieve.

The cost ranges from $900 to $1200 depending on the provider.

Non-invasive lifting procedures

Thermage

Thermage is the most recognised radiofrequency therapy.

Fraxel addresses skin texture and damage from natural aging or sun exposure whereas Thermage uses radiofrequency to provide long-term collagen stimulation to tighten the skin.

It works by inducing thermal damage that raises the temperature in the dermis, which stimulates collagen production in deep layers of the skin tissue. The result is a natural anti-aging process because it is the body doing the work.

It can be used on the face, neck, chest and body. Generally, there is no downtime. Best results are usually seen by six months, as it takes time for collagen tightening to occur.

It is just one treatment and no downtime. You can safely go out straight after a Thermage and the skin keeps gradually improving for six months after having it.

It can be expensive, and cost anywhere between $1500 and $3000 depending on the area being done. It is a good option for people who don't want the dramatic results of surgery but would prefer a more subtle gradual result over time.

Ultratherapy

Ultherapy is also a non-surgical alternative to a facelift. It uses ultrasound technology to kick-start collagen production and tighten skin and counteract signs of aging like skin sagging and wrinkles on the face, neck, and chest as well as drooping of the brow area.

When it comes to non-invasive anti-aging treatments, most experts will agree that the top technologies are radiofrequency, performed with Thermage, and HIFU (high intensity focused ultrasound), performed with Ultherapy.

Beside the types of energy being used to perform the treatment, what are the differences between them? Key points of the face can be targeted with HIFU so prices can vary according to the specific area. A mini HIFU around the eyes can cost $129 whereas the whole face may cost up to $1700.

Tixel

The latest device that cosmetic doctors and dermal therapists around the world have been talking about is the Tixel.

Tixel stimulates collagen production through heat energy. This action is particularly useful for the reduction or complete cure of fine skin lines and wrinkles, as well as skin pigmentations and discolorations. Collagen production by Tixel is also known for treating acne scars, sun damage and uneven skin texture and tone. Increase in collagen and elastin makes skin tighter and firmer.

It is the only machine that can be safely used around the eyes, and after three monthly sessions of Tixel eyelid treatment the tightening and gentle correction of the loose eyelid skin is akin to blepharoplasty (an eyelift discussed in the next chapter)

Tixel has the unique advantage of being far less painful and with a shorter downtime/recovery period. This treatment is ideal for those seeking smoother, more radiant and revitalised looking skin, but who are worried about downtime. The added benefit is that it continues to deliver results that improve over time and can last for several years (as it is your own collagen that produces the effects).

Chapter 20

Surgery of the face

People have so many fears when it comes to cosmetic surgery. Fear of pain, fear of being judged, fear of anaesthesia, fear of scarring. They worry about the outcome, will it look natural? Will it be worth the cost? Fear of uncertainty is a very normal thing and the best thing to do in combating fear is to get as much knowledge as you possibly can and do your research.

I have had three surgeries on my nose. The first was in my 30s as I had a bump removed and it gave me so much more confidence. When I was in my late 40s, however, I had a basal cell carcinoma start to grow right on the end of my nose . . . of all places. It was spreading and had to be removed. I went to a reputable plastic surgeon but he damaged the cartilage so much when he removed it, about five years later my nose began to collapse and I couldn't breathe through it. So I spent a long time investigating who should do the reconstructive surgery. A long time.

I can't emphasise enough how important it is to be confident with your surgeon. The doctor I finally found was wonderful – he saw me three times beforehand to give me the confidence I needed to move forward. It was a long, complicated surgery but now I can breathe again and I am so happy with the result. Surgery can be so daunting and a rhinoplasty has a long downtime – it looks like someone has punched you in the face.

Now I will discuss the different types of face lifts. A facelift is a cosmetic surgical procedure that addresses wrinkles, loose and sagging skin, fat deposits and other visible signs of aging on the face. Surgeons have developed a number of different facelift techniques that focus on different tissue layers.

If your self-confidence is affected by the appearance of sagging skin and non-invasive treatments don't seem to be working, a facelift may be the most effective solution. It is the most comprehensive approach to treating facial sagging caused by aging. It removes the excess skin, tightens the underlying tissues and muscle and then redrapes the skin on the face and neck.

Costs quoted are approximate and cover the surgeon's fees. The costs do not include an anaesthetist's fees or the hospital and theatre costs.

Thread lifts

If you are not quite ready for a facelift but eager to do something this may be the first step for you. Thread lifts are a less invasive procedure that tighten your skin by inserting medical-grade thread material into your face and then 'pulling' your skin up by tightening the thread. The threads have small barbs that are tugged to lift the sagging tissue.

Thread lifts are not as dramatic as a facelift but can provide a visible, natural-looking lift while encouraging the growth of skin-renewing collagen for immediate rejuvenation without surgery or downtime. Thread lifts are ideal for treating skin anywhere on the face, such as the forehead, mouth, jowls or crêpey neck skin. The procedure lasts about 12 to 18 months and is generally undertaken by people in their 40s who are just starting to show signs of facial sagging.

They have very little downtime as they are minimally invasive and they range in cost and start at about $2000 depending on your requirements.

Eye lifts

It might be that you think you need a facelift, however you may only need the amazing results of an eyelift. When people are looking at you, they generally look at your eyes. The two most common types of eye lifts are on the excess skin of the upper eyelid and the lower eyelid grooves.

An upper eyelid lift, also known as upper blepharoplasty, has one of the quickest recovery times and can make a dramatic difference by getting rid of excess skin. If your upper eyelids are saggy or have excess skin, this can make you look tired. Removing this skin can make you look younger, more alert and can show off the sparkle in your eyes. It can be done with a local or twilight anesthetic, you won't need a general and there is a short downtime of approximately five days.

Having skin removed from the lower lid tends to involve longer recovery times. Lower eyelid surgery is for the purpose of removing the fat under the eyes that causes 'bags'.

Both these types of lifts can now be performed with a CO_2 laser. Laser blepharoplasty is a revolutionary procedure that is quickly becoming far more popular than the traditional scalpel method, and for good reason when you consider all of its amazing benefits. There is less risk of infection, less swelling, reduced risk of scarring, and patients seem to have less post-operative pain.

Laser eyelid surgery can range in price from $2000 to $5000 while the traditional method is similar in price depending on the complexity of the patient's requirements.

Brow or forehead lifts

If your eyes are looking tired because of heaviness or sagging of the eyebrows, then a brow lift will be what you need. This can be done in conjunction with an upper eyelid lift if required. The brow lift procedure will stabilise the eyebrow, indirectly improving the upper eyelid position, and will improve the skin causing outer corner hooding in the upper eyelids or any heavy brows that may hang over the eye socket above the eyelids.

It will also soften any deep forehead creases and horizontal frown lines at the top of your nose. Ultimately it will open up your eyes and make you look rejuvenated.

The Endoscopic Brow Lift is the most commonly used technique for this type of procedure as it is much less invasive than previous techniques yet still achieves an equally good result. The procedure includes making a series of very short incisions just behind the hairline. Then, using a special tiny camera and thin instruments, to reposition the muscles and lift underlying tissues of the forehead. It allows for repositioning of the forehead and brow without skin removal.

There is usually very little pain after an endoscopic brow lift, but it is common to feel slight discomfort as well as a sensation of tightness and numbness of the forehead. Swelling and bruising can be common during the first 10 days or so after surgery, but are mostly gone after about two weeks.

The cost is approximately $6000 to $8000.

Mini lift (short scar)

A mini facelift is a modified version of a traditional facelift. In the 'mini' version, a plastic surgeon uses small incisions around your hairline to help lift the lower half of your face to help correct sagging skin. There is less amount of work required to the underlying face muscle.

It is used when your skin has started to show the first signs of aging and is a surgical procedure that tightens the sagging skin and restores the lost chin line. It rejuvenates the lower third of the face and can also be combined with other facial surgeries such as the eyelid lift or neck lift. A mini facelift is most often performed on younger and middle-aged patients who have excess skin in the middle and lower part of the face but who have less pronounced signs of aging.

A mini facelift is conducted via smaller incisions than a traditional facelift and stitches are removed approximately 10 days after surgery. It takes several weeks to fully recover.

They range in cost between $7000 and $12,000.

Neck lift

For many people, the neck is one of the first places where visible signs of aging start to develop. The neck lift can be done as a stand-alone procedure for people who have little facial aging and who require excess skin and fatty tissue to be removed to increase the definition of the jawline. Liposculpture can also be used in this procedure to define the jawline.

The neck lift incisions can vary depending on your case. The surgeon will make a small incision in front of your ear. This incision might be extended around your earlobe and a little behind your ear. Through this incision, your surgeon will pull your platysma muscle and fix it with strong sutures to flatten any visible bands or cords. The remaining skin will be pulled tight to get rid of any skin folds or deep wrinkles on your neck.

You will need to keep your neck still for at least a week following the surgery, although you must also get up and walk around in order to boost your circulation. After the first week you can gradually and gently begin to move your neck.

Costs range from $5000 to $8000.

Mid face

The mid-face facelift targets the nasolabial folds, sagging cheeks and the lower eyelid grooves. If you draw a line from your mouth to the top of your ear canal, everything above this area is considered mid-face.

A mid-face lift can be performed with the traditional facelift as it may not fully treat the upper cheek and lower eyelid areas of the face, which often flatten and lengthen with age. During a mid-face lift, the surgeon makes small incisions behind the hairline. The surgeon then elevates the fat pad in the cheek (called the malar fat pad), providing fullness to the eyes and cheeks. Results are more permanent than those offered by injectables, and recovery from a mid-face lift is quicker than for a traditional facelift.

The cost can range from $7000 to $15,000.

The traditional facelift

A traditional facelift does not lift the mid-face and cheeks. It treats the lower part of the face and neck. You will need both procedures for a fully refreshed look. Traditional facelift only corrects the area below the line from the ear canal to the mouth.

Surgeons have a number of techniques that focus on different tissue layers. A traditional facelift concentrates on the first two layers. This means the underlying tissue layer (the SMAS) is tightened as well as the superficial skin layer for a more natural look that will last longer. Years ago, when people looked unnatural and stretched, only the superficial layer of the skin was tightened.

If you are doing the mid cheek and a traditional facelift, surgery will take approximately four hours. Incisions are made around the front of the ear, behind the earlobe and into the back of the hairline. There will be no scarring if you go to an excellent surgeon. Stitches are removed after seven to 10 days when you can restart normal everyday activities. Strenuous exercise should not be undertaken for about six weeks.

Costs for an SMAS traditional facelift will be between $18,000 and $25,000.

Overseas surgery

Before Covid, approximately 15,000 Australians a year were going overseas for cosmetic surgery. The cheaper prices and exotic locations make cosmetic tourism an attractive option. While Thailand is the most popular, people are undertaking cosmetic surgery procedures in Bali, Dubai, South Korea, India and Mauritius.

The main benefit is cost saving, you can save anywhere between 30% and 80%. You can also recover in private at a beautiful hotel. Many of the medical professionals are trained and also certified, in Western nations, including the UK and the US. Many of the medical centres are accredited by international organisations to prove their excellence, and some are members of the National Institutes of Health.

You cannot ignore the risks, though. It could be difficult to communicate with your doctor and nurses in a foreign country. Medications may be of a poorer quality than what you would receive at home. How can you be sure of the surgeon's skills and experience?

The Australian Society of Plastic Surgeons (ASPS) warned the most common complications arising from cosmetic surgery include scarring, bleeding, infections, fluid accumulation, skin loss, blood clots, numbness, skin discolouration and prolonged swelling. Recovering from these types of complications could be concerning if this were to occur overseas as the follow-up care may not be the same as you would receive in Australia.

Also, antibiotic resistance is a serious problem all over the world, and it could be more widespread in countries where medical tourism is common. Bacterial strains that are resistant to antibiotics can result in complications that include serious infections.

So to finish up here, if you feel that the way you look on the outside doesn't match how you feel on the inside, as many of us do, there are lots of options available to you. Start investigating them and you might be surprised about what you can do. The most important thing is choosing the right plastic surgeon.

Conclusion

There is a lot to unpack from this book. It is basically a summary of the personal development I have done for the last 25 years that has put me in the best physical shape of my life at 55 and the most mentally strong I have ever felt. The best is yet to come for me. I hope it is for you too, no matter what stage of life you may be at.

Where do you go from here? It will depend on a lot of things but it will mostly be decided by what you wish for yourself and how mentally prepared you are to start applying the changes to make it happen. There may be one area of your life that you really want to work on the most, or a couple. Just read those particular chapters again and start to make some small changes. Small changes, consistently practised, can and will change your life.

Become who you want to be and what is right for you at this stage of your life. Not who others want you to be. Be brave, follow your heart and don't worry about what other people will think. Transformation starts with a shift in how you see yourself, who you want to be and who you truly think you are. Listen to your gut because the story you tell yourself every day will ultimately determine who you become both mentally and physically.

I hope that as we move into the future society starts to think differently about aging. What if we were all told today that there has been a medical breakthrough and we can now live until we are 150? How would that change what you think and do today? As we can look and feel healthier for longer, maybe we will start using a different language other than moving into the 'twilight area of our lives' or learning to 'age gracefully'. I know we all have a limited time on this planet, but what's wrong with making it as fun as possible by feeling great, looking better, living a longer life full of energy and enjoying life more generally?

Whatever you do, make sure you tell yourself every day that you matter, you are worth it. Find the reason that is going to put that glint back into your eyes and make your soul light up then fight for it like crazy. Be kind to yourself and to others. Smile at your family, your friends and at someone you don't know. Smile with your eyes and with your soul. It will take years off your face and add years to your life.

Lyndal

x

Acknowledgements

The people who are of the greatest importance in our lives are the ones that know us completely, with all our imperfections, and yet still believe we are capable of anything. They not only encourage you to chase your dreams, they believe wholeheartedly that you will get there. They help you to be brave and have courage, pick you up when you fall and help you to keep going.

My parents are these people for me. Annmaree and John Dwyer, a couple of Broken Hill rock stars. They have a love story of more than 60 years and are the best parents a girl could wish for.

To my husband and partner in life, Gary, thank you for believing I can accomplish anything. Anytime I have started down a new road your unquestioning support has helped me get there and for this I am so grateful. Thank you for your patience while I disappeared for hours on end and for the endless love you give to our family.

I am also lucky to have a someone I can call "my person". That someone who has been my friend forever, knows my "deepest and darkest", and loves me anyway. That someone who shares a lifetime of memories with me. Who has laughed with me until we cried so many times I can't remember. That someone who has given me the advice I needed to hear at exactly the time I needed to hear it. My sister from another mister, George. This book wouldn't have happened without you.

Very occasionally you happen across someone who changes your life in a way that you didn't think was possible. The topic of this book has always been a passion of mine, however I really questioned whether it would be possible to write a book at all, let alone on such a big and diverse subject. Andrew Griffiths gave me the tools I needed to work through all my doubts. The amount of knowledge and small business experience Andrew brings to the table is extraordinary. Thank you so much Andrew for your continual encouragement, guidance, for your belief in me, but most of all for your friendship.

www.ingramcontent.com/pod-product-compliance
Lightning Source LLC
Chambersburg PA
CBHW032054020426
42335CB00011B/341